THE VEGETARIAN DIET
FOR MEN
Cookbook

BONUS: The Best Exercises to **SCULP** your Body!

The Best **100 Recipes** to Stay **FIT**!
Sculpt Your Abs Before Summer
with the Healthiest **Plant-Based Meals**!

By
Jocelyn Grant

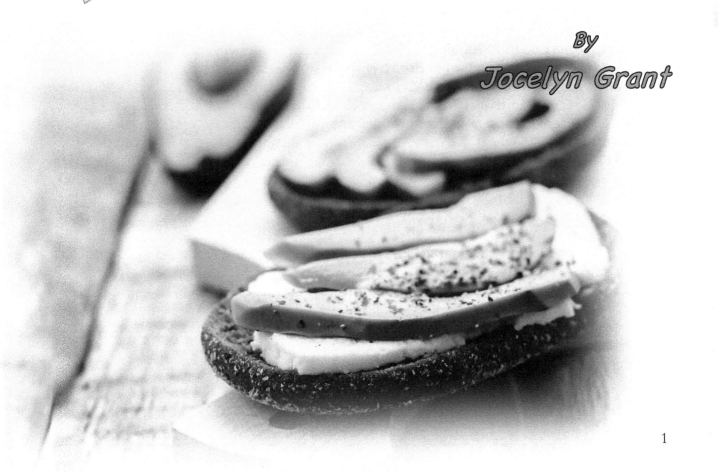

Table of Contents

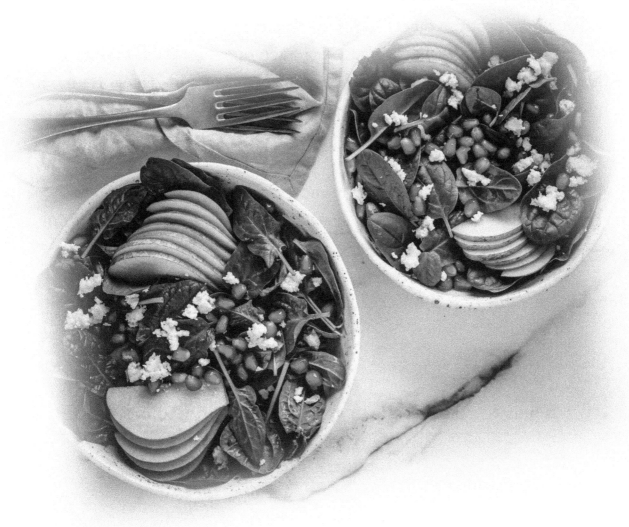

Introduction

In the last years, people are concerned about eating healthy foods to provide the right nutrients to the body. Moreover, they are interested in eating meals that are no full of preservatives or additives. It is essential eat healthy and stay fit to prevent pathologies and feel full of energy!
Wouldn't it be great if you could eat healthy food without additives and feel fit?

Luckily there is a solution: The Vegetarian diet!

Eating Plant-based foods you can resolve all your problems!
Moreover, the vegetarian diet is suitable for everyone: **children**, **people over 50**, **athletes** and **women**. However, there is a specific people category that in my opinion should eat Vegetarian diet absolutely: **MEN**!

The Vegetarian diet allows you to get the right amount of nutrients and follow a meal plan that makes you light and fit; moreover, due to high proteins foods, this diet allows the muscle's body to growth well and <u>**it is perfect for men**</u>!

Whit more than the best **100 Vegetarian Recipes**, in this book you will find also the best exercises to **SCULPT** your body to the **TOP**!

Ready to discover the best 100 Vegetarian Recipes?

<u>LET'S GO!</u>

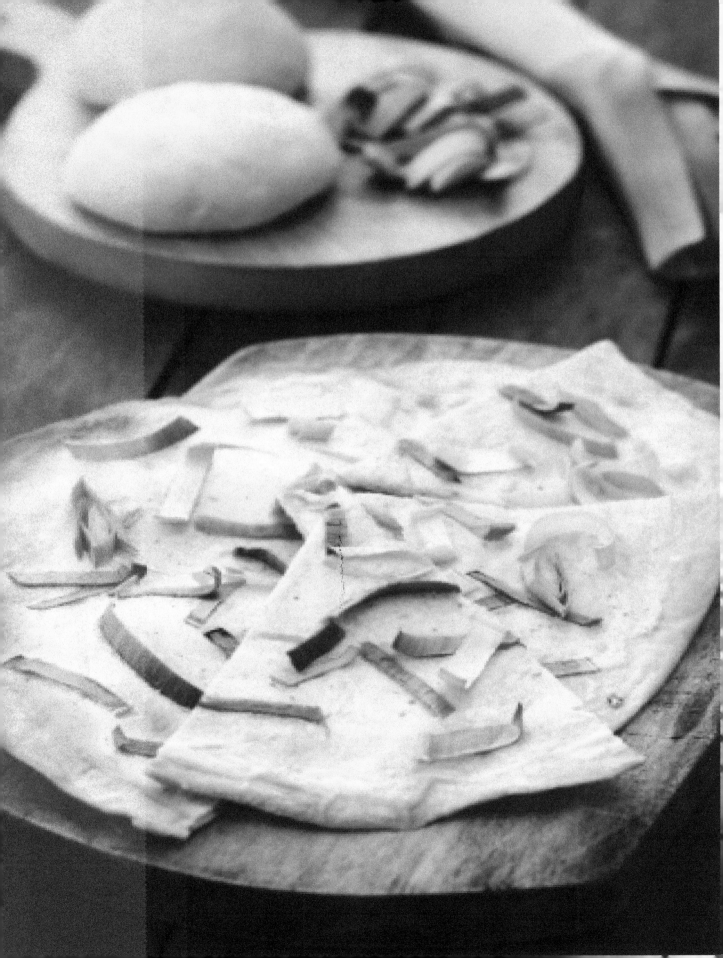

Chapter 1. BREAKFAST AND SNACKS

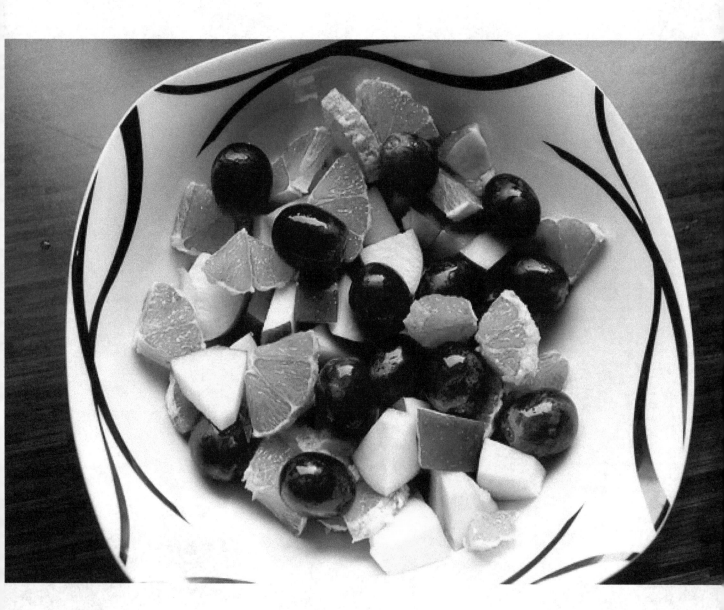

1) ITALIAN MUSHROOM AND SPINACH CHICKPEA OMELETTE

Preparation Time: 25 minutes | | **Servings:** 4

Ingredients:

- ✓ 1 cup chickpea flour
- ✓ ½ tsp onion powder
- ✓ ½ tsp garlic powder
- ✓ ¼ tsp white pepper
- ✓ 1/3 cup nutritional yeast
- ✓ ½ tsp baking soda
- ✓ 1 green bell pepper, chopped
- ✓ 3 scallions, chopped
- ✓ 1 cup sautéed button mushrooms
- ✓ ½ cup chopped fresh spinach
- ✓ 1 cup halved cherry tomatoes
- ✓ 1 tbsp fresh parsley leaves

Directions:

❖ In a medium bowl, mix the chickpea flour, onion powder, garlic powder, white pepper, nutritional yeast, and baking soda until well combined. Heat a medium skillet over medium heat and add a quarter of the batter. Swirl the pan to spread the batter across the pan. Scatter a quarter each of the bell pepper, scallions, mushrooms, and spinach on top and cook until the bottom part of the omelet sets, 1-2 minutes.

❖ Carefully flip the omelet and cook the other side until set and golden brown. Transfer the omelet to a plate and make the remaining omelets. Serve the omelet with the tomatoes and garnish with the parsley leaves

2) EXOTIC COCONUT-RASPBERRY PANCAKES

Preparation Time: 25 minutes | | **Servings:** 4

Ingredients:

- ✓ 2 tbsp flax seed powder
- ✓ ½ cup coconut milk
- ✓ ¼ cup fresh raspberries, mashed
- ✓ ½ cup oat flour
- ✓ 1 tsp baking soda
- ✓ A pinch salt
- ✓ 1 tbsp coconut sugar
- ✓ 2 tbsp pure date syrup
- ✓ ½ tsp cinnamon powder
- ✓ 2 tbsp unsweetened coconut flakes
- ✓ 2 tsp plant butter
- ✓ Fresh raspberries for garnishing

Directions:

❖ In a medium bowl, mix the flax seed powder with the 6 tbsp water and thicken for 5 minutes. Mix in coconut milk and raspberries. Add the oat flour, baking soda, salt, coconut sugar, date syrup, and cinnamon powder. Fold in the coconut flakes until well combined.

❖ Working in batches, melt a quarter of the butter in a non-stick skillet and add ¼ cup of the batter. Cook until set beneath and golden brown, 2 minutes. Flip the pancake and cook on the other side until set and golden brown, 2 minutes. Transfer to a plate and make the remaining pancakes using the rest of the ingredients in the same proportions. Garnish the pancakes with some raspberries and serve warm

3) ENGLISH BLUEBERRY-CHIA PUDDING

Preparation Time: 5 minutes + chilling time | | **Servings:** 2

Ingredients:

- ✓ ¾ cup coconut milk
- ✓ ½ tsp vanilla extract
- ✓ ½ cup blueberries
- ✓ 2 tbsp chia seeds
- ✓ Chopped walnuts to garnish

Directions:

❖ In a blender, pour the coconut milk, vanilla extract, and half of the blueberries. Process the ingredients at high speed until the blueberries have incorporated into the liquid.

❖ Open the blender and mix in the chia seeds. Share the mixture into two breakfast jars, cover, and refrigerate for 4 hours to allow the mixture to gel. Garnish the pudding with the remaining blueberries and walnuts. Serve immediately

4) EASY POTATO AND CAULIFLOWER BROWNS

Preparation Time: 35 minutes

Servings: 4

Ingredients:

- ✓ 3 tbsp flax seed powder
- ✓ 2 large potatoes, shredded
- ✓ 1 big head cauliflower, riced
- ✓ ½ white onion, grated
- ✓ Salt and black pepper to taste
- ✓ 4 tbsp plant butter

Directions:

- ❖ In a medium bowl, mix the flaxseed powder and 9 tbsp water. Allow thickening for 5 minutes for the vegan "flax egg." Add the potatoes, cauliflower, onion, salt, and black pepper to the vegan "flax egg" and mix until well combined. Allow sitting for 5 minutes to thicken.
- ❖ Working in batches, melt 1 tbsp of plant butter in a non-stick skillet and add 4 scoops of the hashbrown mixture to the skillet. Make sure to have 1 to 2-inch intervals between each scoop.
- ❖ Use the spoon to flatten the batter and cook until compacted and golden brown on the bottom part, 2 minutes. Flip the hashbrowns and cook further for 2 minutes or until the vegetable cook and is golden brown. Transfer to a paper-towel-lined plate to drain grease. Make the remaining hashbrowns using the remaining ingredients. Serve warm

5) QUICK PISTACHIOS-PUMPKIN CAKE

Preparation Time: 70 minutes

Servings: 4

Ingredients:

- ✓ 2 tbsp flaxseed powder
- ✓ 3 tbsp vegetable oil
- ✓ ¾ cup canned pumpkin puree
- ✓ ½ cup pure corn syrup
- ✓ 3 tbsp pure date sugar
- ✓ 1 ½ cups whole-wheat flour
- ✓ ½ tsp cinnamon powder
- ✓ ½ tsp baking powder
- ✓ ¼ tsp cloves powder
- ✓ ½ tsp allspice powder
- ✓ ½ tsp nutmeg powder
- ✓ 2 tbsp chopped pistachios

Directions:

- ❖ Preheat the oven to 350 F and lightly coat an 8 x 4-inch loaf pan with cooking spray. In a bowl, mix the flax seed powder with 6 tbsp water and allow thickening for 5 minutes to make the vegan "flax egg."
- ❖ In a bowl, whisk the vegetable oil, pumpkin puree, corn syrup, date sugar, and vegan "flax egg." In another bowl, mix the flour, cinnamon powder, baking powder, cloves powder, allspice powder, and nutmeg powder. Add this mixture to the wet batter and mix until well combined. Pour the batter into the loaf pan, sprinkle the pistachios on top, and gently press the nuts onto the batter to stick.
- ❖ Bake in the oven for 50-55 minutes or until a toothpick inserted into the cake comes out clean. Remove the cake onto a wire rack, allow cooling, slice, and serve

6) SPECIAL BELL PEPPER WITH SCRAMBLED TOFU

Preparation Time: 20 minutes

Servings: 4

Ingredients:

- ✓ 2 tbsp plant butter, for frying
- ✓ 1 (14 oz) pack firm tofu, crumbled
- ✓ 1 red bell pepper, chopped
- ✓ 1 green bell pepper, chopped
- ✓ 1 tomato, finely chopped
- ✓ 2 tbsp chopped fresh green onions
- ✓ Salt and black pepper to taste
- ✓ 1 tsp turmeric powder
- ✓ 1 tsp Creole seasoning
- ✓ ½ cup chopped baby kale
- ✓ ¼ cup grated plant-based Parmesan

Directions:

- ❖ Melt the plant butter in a skillet over medium heat and add the tofu. Cook with occasional stirring until the tofu is light golden brown while, making sure not to break the tofu into tiny bits but to have scrambled egg resemblance, 5 minutes.
- ❖ Stir in the bell peppers, tomato, green onions, salt, black pepper, turmeric powder, and Creole seasoning. Sauté until the vegetables soften, 5 minutes. Mix in the kale to wilt, 3 minutes and then half of the plant-based Parmesan cheese.
- ❖ Allow melting for 1 to 2 minutes and then turn the heat off. Top with the remaining cheese and serve warm

7) TRADITIONAL FRENCH TOAST

Preparation Time: 20 minutes		Servings: 2

Ingredients:

- ✓ 1 tbsp ground flax seeds
- ✓ 1 cup coconut milk
- ✓ 1/2 tsp vanilla paste
- ✓ A pinch of sea salt
- ✓ A pinch of grated nutmeg
- ✓ 1/2 tsp ground cinnamon
- ✓ 1/4 tsp ground cloves
- ✓ 1 tbsp agave syrup
- ✓ 4 slices bread

Directions:

- ❖ In a mixing bowl, thoroughly combine the flax seeds, coconut milk, vanilla, salt, nutmeg, cinnamon, cloves and agave syrup.
- ❖ Dredge each slice of bread into the milk mixture until well coated on all sides.
- ❖ Preheat an electric griddle to medium heat and lightly oil it with a nonstick cooking spray.
- ❖ Cook each slice of bread on the preheated griddle for about 3 minutes per side until golden brown.
- ❖ Enjoy

8) CRISPY FRYBREAD WITH PEANUT BUTTER AND JAM

Preparation Time: 20 minutes		Servings: 3

Ingredients:

- ✓ 1 cup all-purpose flour
- ✓ 1/2 tsp baking powder
- ✓ 1/2 tsp sea salt
- ✓ 1 tsp coconut sugar
- ✓ 1/2 cup warm water
- ✓ 3 tsp olive oil
- ✓ 3 tbsp peanut butter
- ✓ 3 tbsp raspberry jam

Directions:

- ❖ Thoroughly combine the flour, baking powder, salt and sugar. Gradually add in the water until the dough comes together.
- ❖ Divide the dough into three balls; flatten each ball to create circles.
- ❖ Heat 1 tsp of the olive oil in a frying pan over a moderate flame. Fry the first bread for about 9 minutes or until golden brown. Repeat with the remaining oil and dough.
- ❖ Serve the frybread with the peanut butter and raspberry jam. Enjoy

9) EASY PUDDING WITH SULTANAS ON CIABATTA BREAD

Preparation Time: 2 hours 10 minutes		Servings: 4

Ingredients:

- ✓ 2 cups coconut milk, unsweetened
- ✓ 1/2 cup agave syrup
- ✓ 1 tbsp coconut oil
- ✓ 1/2 tsp vanilla essence
- ✓ 1/2 tsp ground cardamom
- ✓ 1/4 tsp ground cloves
- ✓ 1/2 tsp ground cinnamon
- ✓ 1/4 tsp Himalayan salt
- ✓ 3/4 pound stale ciabatta bread, cubed
- ✓ 1/2 cup sultana raisins

Directions:

- ❖ In a mixing bowl, combine the coconut milk, agave syrup, coconut oil, vanilla, cardamom, ground cloves, cinnamon and Himalayan salt.
- ❖ Add the bread cubes to the custard mixture and stir to combine well. Fold in the sultana raisins and allow it to rest for about 1 hour on a counter.
- ❖ Then, spoon the mixture into a lightly oiled casserole dish.
- ❖ Bake in the preheated oven at 350 degrees F for about 1 hour or until the top is golden brown.
- ❖ Place the bread pudding on a wire rack for 10 minutes before slicing and serving

10) VEGAN FRIENDLY BANH MI

Preparation Time: 35 minutes | | **Servings:** 4

Ingredients:

- ✓ 1/2 cup rice vinegar
- ✓ 1/4 cup water
- ✓ 1/4 cup white sugar
- ✓ 2 carrots, cut into 1/16-inch-thick matchsticks
- ✓ 1/2 cup white (daikon) radish, cut into 1/16-inch-thick matchsticks
- ✓ 1 white onion, thinly sliced
- ✓ 2 tbsp olive oil
- ✓ 12 ounces firm tofu, cut into sticks
- ✓ 1/4 cup vegan mayonnaise
- ✓ 1 ½ tbsp soy sauce
- ✓ 2 cloves garlic, minced
- ✓ 1/4 cup fresh parsley, chopped
- ✓ Kosher salt and ground black pepper, to taste
- ✓ 2 standard French baguettes, cut into four pieces
- ✓ 4 tbsp fresh cilantro, chopped
- ✓ 4 lime wedges

Directions:

- ❖ Bring the rice vinegar, water and sugar to a boil and stir until the sugar has dissolved, about 1 minute. Allow it to cool.
- ❖ Pour the cooled vinegar mixture over the carrot, daikon radish and onion; allow the vegetables to marinate for at least 30 minutes.
- ❖ While the vegetables are marinating, heat the olive oil in a frying pan over medium-high heat. Once hot, add the tofu and sauté for 8 minutes, stirring occasionally to promote even cooking.
- ❖ Then, mix the mayo, soy sauce, garlic, parsley, salt and ground black pepper in a small bowl.
- ❖ Slice each piece of the baguette in half the long way Then, toast the baguette halves under the preheated broiler for about 3 minutes.
- ❖ To assemble the banh mi sandwiches, spread each half of the toasted baguette with the mayonnaise mixture; fill the cavity of the bottom half of the bread with the fried tofu sticks, marinated vegetables and cilantro leaves.
- ❖ Lastly, squeeze the lime wedges over the filling and top with the other half of the baguette. Enjoy

11) EASY BREAKFAST NUTTY OATMEAL MUFFINS

Preparation Time: 30 minutes | | **Servings:** 9

Ingredients:

- ✓ 1 ½ cups rolled oats
- ✓ 1/2 cup shredded coconut, unsweetened
- ✓ 3/4 tsp baking powder
- ✓ 1/4 tsp salt
- ✓ 1/4 tsp vanilla extract
- ✓ 1/4 tsp coconut extract
- ✓ 1/4 tsp grated nutmeg
- ✓ 1/2 tsp cardamom
- ✓ 3/4 cup coconut milk
- ✓ 1/3 cup canned pumpkin
- ✓ 1/4 cup agave syrup
- ✓ 1/4 cup golden raisins
- ✓ 1/4 cup pecans, chopped

Directions:

- ❖ Begin by preheating your oven to 360 degrees F. Spritz a muffin tin with a nonstick cooking oil.
- ❖ In a mixing bowl, thoroughly combine all the ingredients, except for the raisins and pecans.
- ❖ Fold in the raisins and pecans and scrape the batter into the prepared muffin tin.
- ❖ Bake your muffins for about 25 minutes or until the top is set. Enjoy

12) SPECIAL Smoothie Bowl of Raspberry and Chia

Preparation Time: 10 minutes | | **Servings:** 2

Ingredients:

- ✓ 1 cup coconut milk
- ✓ 2 small-sized bananas, peeled
- ✓ 1 ½ cups raspberries, fresh or frozen
- ✓ 2 dates, pitted
- ✓ 1 tbsp coconut flakes
- ✓ 1 tbsp pepitas
- ✓ 2 tbsp chia seeds

Directions:

- ❖ In your blender or food processor, mix the coconut milk with the bananas, raspberries and dates.
- ❖ Process until creamy and smooth. Divide the smoothie between two bowls.
- ❖ Top each smoothie bowl with the coconut flakes, pepitas and chia seeds. Enjoy

13) ORIGINAL BREAKFAST OATS WITH WALNUTS AND CURRANTS

Preparation Time: 10 minutes		Servings: 2

Ingredients:

- ✓ 1 cup water
- ✓ 1 ½ cups oat milk
- ✓ 1 ½ cups rolled oats
- ✓ A pinch of salt
- ✓ A pinch of grated nutmeg
- ✓ 1/4 tsp cardamom
- ✓ 1 handful walnuts, roughly chopped
- ✓ 4 tbsp dried currants

Directions:

- ❖ In a deep saucepan, bring the water and milk to a rolling boil. Add in the oats, cover the saucepan and turn the heat to medium.
- ❖ Add in the salt, nutmeg and cardamom. Continue to cook for about 12 to 13 minutes more, stirring occasionally.
- ❖ Spoon the mixture into serving bowls; top with walnuts and currants. Enjoy

14) SWEET APPLESAUCE PANCAKES WITH COCONUT

Preparation Time: 50 minutes		Servings: 8

Ingredients:

- ✓ 1 ¼ cups whole-wheat flour
- ✓ 1 tsp baking powder
- ✓ 1/4 tsp sea salt
- ✓ 1/2 tsp coconut sugar
- ✓ 1/4 tsp ground cloves
- ✓ 1/4 tsp ground cardamom
- ✓ 1/2 tsp ground cinnamon
- ✓ 3/4 cup oat milk
- ✓ 1/2 cup applesauce, unsweetened
- ✓ 2 tbsp coconut oil
- ✓ 8 tbsp coconut, shredded
- ✓ 8 tbsp pure maple syrup

Directions:

- ❖ In a mixing bowl, thoroughly combine the flour, baking powder, salt, sugar and spices. Gradually add in the milk and applesauce.
- ❖ Heat a frying pan over a moderately high flame and add a small amount of the coconut oil.
- ❖ Once hot, pour the batter into the frying pan. Cook for approximately 3 minutes until the bubbles form; flip it and cook on the other side for 3 minutes longer until browned on the underside. Repeat with the remaining oil and batter.
- ❖ Serve with shredded coconut and maple syrup. Enjoy

15) LOVELY VEGGIE PANINI

Preparation Time: 30 minutes		Servings: 4

Ingredients:

- ✓ 1 tbsp olive oil
- ✓ 1 cup sliced button mushrooms
- ✓ Salt and black pepper to taste
- ✓ 1 ripe avocado, sliced
- ✓ 2 tbsp freshly squeezed lemon juice
- ✓ 1 tbsp chopped parsley
- ✓ ½ tsp pure maple syrup
- ✓ 8 slices whole-wheat ciabatta
- ✓ 4 oz sliced plant-based Parmesan

Directions:

- ❖ Heat the olive oil in a medium skillet over medium heat and sauté the mushrooms until softened, 5 minutes. Season with salt and black pepper. Turn the heat off.
- ❖ Preheat a panini press to medium heat, 3 to 5 minutes. Mash the avocado in a medium bowl and mix in the lemon juice, parsley, and maple syrup. Spread the mixture on 4 bread slices, divide the mushrooms and plant-based Parmesan cheese on top.
- ❖ Cover with the other bread slices and brush the top with olive oil. Grill the sandwiches one after another in the heated press until golden brown, and the cheese is melted.
- ❖ Serve

16) TASTY Cheddar Grits and Soy Chorizo

Preparation Time: 25 minutes		**Servings:** 6

Ingredients:

- ✓ 1 cup quick-cooking grits
- ✓ ½ cup grated plant-based cheddar
- ✓ 2 tbsp peanut butter
- ✓ 1 cup soy chorizo, chopped
- ✓ 1 cup corn kernels
- ✓ 2 cups vegetable broth

Directions:

- ❖ Preheat oven to 380 F.
- ❖ Pour the broth in a pot and bring to a boil over medium heat. Stir in salt and grits. Lower the heat and cook until the grits are thickened, stirring often. Turn the heat off, put in the plant-based cheddar cheese, peanut butter, soy chorizo, and corn and mix well.
- ❖ Spread the mixture into a greased baking dish and bake for 45 minutes until slightly puffed and golden brown. Serve right away

17) NEW VANILLA CREPES AND BERRY CREAM COMPOTE TOPPING

Preparation Time: 35 minutes		**Servings:** 4

Ingredients:

- ✓ For the berry cream:
- ✓ 2 tbsp plant butter
- ✓ 2 tbsp pure date sugar
- ✓ 1 tsp vanilla extract
- ✓ ½ cup fresh blueberries
- ✓ ½ cup fresh raspberries
- ✓ ½ cup whipped coconut cream
- ✓ For the crepes:
- ✓ 2 tbsp flax seed powder
- ✓ 1 tsp vanilla extract
- ✓ 1 tsp pure date sugar
- ✓ ¼ tsp salt
- ✓ 2 cups almond flour
- ✓ 1 ½ cups almond milk
- ✓ 1 ½ cups water
- ✓ 3 tbsp plant butter for frying

Directions:

- ❖ Melt butter in a pot over low heat and mix in the date sugar, and vanilla. Cook until the sugar melts and then toss in berries. Allow softening for 2-3 minutes. Set aside to cool.
- ❖ In a medium bowl, mix the flax seed powder with 6 tbsp water and allow to thicken for 5 minutes to make the vegan "flax egg." Whisk in vanilla, date sugar, and salt. Pour in a quarter cup of almond flour and whisk, then a quarter cup of almond milk, and mix until no lumps remain. Repeat the mixing process with the remaining almond flour and almond milk in the same quantities until exhausted.
- ❖ Mix in 1 cup of water until the mixture is runny like that of pancakes and add the remaining water until it is lighter. Brush a large non-stick skillet with some butter and place over medium heat to melt. Pour 1 tbsp of the batter into the pan and swirl the skillet quickly and all around to coat the pan with the batter. Cook until the batter is dry and golden brown beneath, about 30 seconds.
- ❖ Use a spatula to carefully flip the crepe and cook the other side until golden brown too. Fold the crepe onto a plate and set aside. Repeat making more crepes with the remaining batter until exhausted. Plate the crepes, top with the whipped coconut cream and the berry compote. Serve immediately

18) ORIGINAL BREAKFAST NAAN BREAD WITH MANGO JAM

Preparation Time: 40 minutes

Servings: 4

Ingredients:

- ¾ cup almond flour
- 1 tsp salt + extra for sprinkling
- 1 tsp baking powder
- 1/3 cup olive oil
- 2 cups boiling water
- 2 tbsp plant butter for frying
- 4 cups heaped chopped mangoes
- 1 cup pure maple syrup
- 1 lemon, juiced
- A pinch of saffron powder
- 1 tsp cardamom powder

Directions:

- In a large bowl, mix the almond flour, salt, and baking powder. Mix in the olive oil and boiling water until smooth, thick batter forms. Allow the dough to rise for 5 minutes. Form balls out of the dough, place each on a baking paper, and use your hands to flatten the dough.
- Working in batches, melt the plant butter in a large skillet and fry the dough on both sides until set and golden brown on each side, 4 minutes per bread. Transfer to a plate and set aside for serving.
- Add mangoes, maple syrup, lemon juice, and 3 tbsp water in a pot and cook until boiling, 5 minutes. Mix in saffron and cardamom powders and cook further over low heat until the mangoes soften. Mash the mangoes with the back of the spoon until relatively smooth with little chunks of mangoes in a jam.
- Cool completely. Spoon the jam into sterilized jars and serve with the naan bread

19) SPECIAL Crispy Corn Cakes

Preparation Time: 35 minutes

Servings: 4

Ingredients:

- 1 tbsp flaxseed powder
- 2 cups yellow cornmeal
- 1 tsp salt
- 2 tsp baking powder
- 4 tbsp olive oil
- 1 cup tofu mayonnaise for serving

Directions:

- In a bowl, mix the flax seed powder with 3 tbsp water and allow thickening for 5 minutes to form the vegan "flax egg." Mix in 1 cup of water and then whisk in the cornmeal, salt, and baking powder until soup texture forms but not watery.
- Heat a quarter of the olive oil in a griddle pan and pour in a quarter of the batter. Cook until set and golden brown beneath, 3 minutes. Flip the cake and cook the other side until set and golden brown too. Plate the cake and make three more with the remaining oil and batter.
- Top the cakes with some tofu mayonnaise before serving

20) EXOTIC CHIA COCONUT PUDDING

Preparation Time: 5 minutes+ cooling time

Servings: 4

Ingredients:

- 1 cup coconut milk
- ½ tsp vanilla extract
- 3 tbsp chia seeds
- ½ cup granola
- 2/3 cup chopped sweet nectarine

Directions:

- In a medium bowl, mix the coconut milk, vanilla, and chia seeds until well combined. Divide the mixture between 4 breakfast cups and refrigerate for at least 4 hours to allow the mixture to gel.
- Top with the granola and nectarine. Serve

21) ITALIAN CHOCOLATE AND CARROT BREAD WITH RAISINS

Preparation Time: 75 minutes		Servings: 4

Ingredients:

- ✓ 1 ½ cup whole-wheat flour
- ✓ ¼ cup almond flour
- ✓ ¼ tsp salt
- ✓ ¼ tsp cloves powder
- ✓ ¼ tsp cayenne pepper
- ✓ 1 tbsp cinnamon powder
- ✓ ½ tsp nutmeg powder
- ✓ 1 ½ tsp baking powder
- ✓ 2 tbsp flax seed powder
- ✓ ½ cup pure date sugar

- ✓ ¼ cup pure maple syrup
- ✓ ¾ tsp almond extract
- ✓ 1 tbsp grated lemon zest
- ✓ ½ cup unsweetened applesauce
- ✓ ¼ cup olive oil
- ✓ 4 carrots, shredded
- ✓ 3 tbsp unsweetened chocolate chips
- ✓ 2/3 cup black raisins

Directions:

- ❖ Preheat oven to 375 F and line a loaf tin with baking paper. In a bowl, mix all the flours, salt, cloves powder, cayenne pepper, cinnamon powder, nutmeg powder, and baking powder.
- ❖ In another bowl, mix the flax seed powder, 6 tbsp water, and allow thickening for 5 minutes. Mix in the date sugar, maple syrup, almond extract, lemon zest, applesauce, and olive oil. Combine both mixtures until smooth and fold in the carrots, chocolate chips, and raisins.
- ❖ Pour the mixture into a loaf pan and bake in the oven until golden brown on top or a toothpick inserted into the bread comes out clean, 45-50 minutes. Remove from the oven, transfer the bread onto a wire rack to cool, slice, and serve

22) FRENCH TOASTS TROPICAL STYLE

Preparation Time: 55 minutes		Servings: 4

Ingredients:

- ✓ 2 tbsp flax seed powder
- ✓ 1 ½ cups unsweetened almond milk
- ✓ ½ cup almond flour
- ✓ 2 tbsp maple syrup + extra for drizzling
- ✓ 2 pinches of salt

- ✓ ½ tbsp cinnamon powder
- ✓ ½ tsp fresh lemon zest
- ✓ 1 tbsp fresh pineapple juice
- ✓ 8 whole-grain bread slices

Directions:

- ❖ Preheat the oven to 400 F and lightly grease a roasting rack with olive oil. Set aside.
- ❖ In a medium bowl, mix the flax seed powder with 6 tbsp water and allow thickening for 5 to 10 minutes. Whisk in the almond milk, almond flour, maple syrup, salt, cinnamon powder, lemon zest, and pineapple juice. Soak the bread on both sides in the almond milk mixture and allow sitting on a plate for 2 to 3 minutes.
- ❖ Heat a large skillet over medium heat and place the bread in the pan. Cook until golden brown on the bottom side. Flip the bread and cook further until golden brown on the other side, 4 minutes in total. Transfer to a plate, drizzle some maple syrup on top and serve immediately

23) SPECIAL CREPES WITH MUSHROOM

Preparation Time: 25 minutes		Servings: 4

Ingredients:

- ✓ 1 cup whole-wheat flour
- ✓ 1 tsp onion powder
- ✓ ½ tsp baking soda
- ✓ ¼ tsp salt
- ✓ 1 cup pressed, crumbled tofu
- ✓ ⅓ cup plant-based milk

- ✓ ¼ cup lemon juice
- ✓ 2 tbsp extra-virgin olive oil
- ✓ ½ cup finely chopped mushrooms
- ✓ ½ cup finely chopped onion
- ✓ 2 cups collard greens

Directions:

- ❖ Combine the flour, onion powder, baking soda, and salt in a bowl. Blitz the tofu, milk, lemon juice, and oil in a food processor over high speed for 30 seconds. Pour over the flour mixture and mix to combine well. Add in the mushrooms, onion, and collard greens.
- ❖ Heat a skillet and grease with cooking spray. Lower the heat and spread a ladleful of the batter across the surface of the skillet. Cook for 4 minutes on both sides or until set. Remove to a plate. Repeat the process until no batter is left, greasing with a little more oil, if needed. Serve

24) SPECIAL FRENCH TOAST WITH CINNAMON-BANANA

Preparation Time: 25 minutes		Servings: 3

Ingredients:

- ✓ 1/3 cup coconut milk
- ✓ 1/2 cup banana, mashed
- ✓ 2 tbsp besan (chickpea flour)
- ✓ 1/2 tsp baking powder
- ✓ 1/2 tsp vanilla paste
- ✓ A pinch of sea salt
- ✓ 1 tbsp agave syrup
- ✓ 1/2 tsp ground allspice
- ✓ A pinch of grated nutmeg
- ✓ 6 slices day-old sourdough bread
- ✓ 2 bananas, sliced
- ✓ 2 tbsp brown sugar
- ✓ 1 tsp ground cinnamon

Directions:

- ❖ To make the batter, thoroughly combine the coconut milk, mashed banana, besan, baking powder, vanilla, salt, agave syrup, allspice and nutmeg.
- ❖ Dredge each slice of bread into the batter until well coated on all sides.
- ❖ Preheat an electric griddle to medium heat and lightly oil it with a nonstick cooking spray.
- ❖ Cook each slice of bread on the preheated griddle for about 3 minutes per side until golden brown.
- ❖ Garnish the French toast with the bananas, brown sugar and cinnamon. Enjoy

25) INDIAN AUTHENTIC ROTI

Preparation Time: 30 minutes		Servings: 5

Ingredients:

- ✓ 2 cups bread flour
- ✓ 1 tsp baking powder
- ✓ 1/2 tsp salt
- ✓ 3/4 warm water
- ✓ 1 cup vegetable oil, for frying

Directions:

- ❖ Thoroughly combine the flour, baking powder and salt in a mixing bowl. Gradually add in the water until the dough comes together.
- ❖ Divide the dough into five balls; flatten each ball to create circles.
- ❖ Heat the olive oil in a frying pan over a moderately high flame. Fry the first bread, turning it over to promote even cooking; fry it for about 10 minutes or until golden brown.
- ❖ Repeat with the remaining dough. Transfer each roti to a paper towel-lined plate to drain the excess oil.
- ❖ Enjoy

26) TYPICAL CHIA CHOCOLATE PUDDING

Preparation Time: 10 minutes + chilling time		Servings: 4

Ingredients:

- ✓ 4 tbsp unsweetened cocoa powder
- ✓ 4 tbsp maple syrup
- ✓ 1 2/3 cups coconut milk
- ✓ A pinch of grated nutmeg
- ✓ A pinch of ground cloves
- ✓ 1/2 tsp ground cinnamon
- ✓ 1/2 cup chia seeds

Directions:

- ❖ Add the cocoa powder, maple syrup, milk and spices to a bowl and stir until everything is well incorporated.
- ❖ Add in the chia seeds and stir again to combine well. Spoon the mixture into four jars, cover and place in your refrigerator overnight.
- ❖ On the actual day, stir with a spoon and serve. Enjoy

Chapter 2. LUNCH

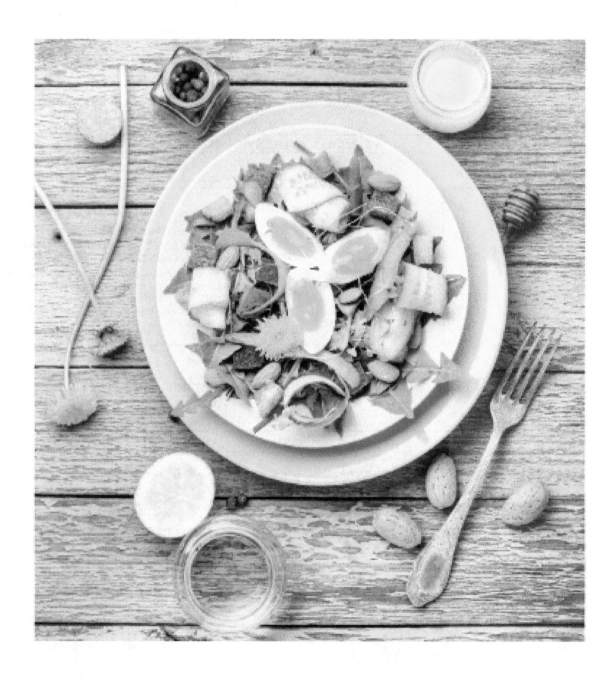

27) WHITE WINE AND LEMON BRAISED ARTICHOKES

Preparation Time: 35 minutes		Servings: 4

Ingredients:

- ✓ 1 large lemon, freshly squeezed
- ✓ 1 ½ pounds artichokes, trimmed, tough outer leaves and chokes removed
- ✓ 2 tbsp mint leaves, finely chopped
- ✓ 2 tbsp cilantro leaves, finely chopped
- ✓ 2 tbsp basil leaves, finely chopped
- ✓ 2 cloves garlic, minced
- ✓ 1/4 cup dry white wine
- ✓ 1/4 cup extra-virgin olive oil, plus more for drizzling
- ✓ Sea salt and freshly ground black pepper, to taste

Directions:

- ❖ Fill a bowl with water and add in the lemon juice. Place the cleaned artichokes in the bowl, keeping them completely submerged.
- ❖ In another small bowl, thoroughly combine the herbs and garlic. Rub your artichokes with the herb mixture.
- ❖ Pour the wine and olive oil in a saucepan; add the artichokes to the saucepan. Turn the heat to a simmer and continue to cook, covered, for about 30 minutes until the artichokes are crisp-tender.
- ❖ To serve, drizzle the artichokes with the cooking juices, season them with the salt and black pepper and enjoy

28) SUPER ROASTED CARROTS WITH HERBS

Preparation Time: 25 minute		Servings: 4

Ingredients:

- ✓ 2 pounds carrots, trimmed and halved lengthwise
- ✓ 4 tbsp olive oil
- ✓ 1 tsp granulated garlic
- ✓ 1 tsp paprika
- ✓ Sea salt and freshly ground black pepper
- ✓ 2 tbsp fresh cilantro, chopped
- ✓ 2 tbsp fresh parsley, chopped
- ✓ 2 tbsp fresh chives, chopped

Directions:

- ❖ Start by preheating your oven to 400 degrees F.
- ❖ Toss the carrots with the olive oil, granulated garlic, paprika, salt and black pepper. Arrange them in a single layer on a parchment-lined roasting sheet.
- ❖ Roast the carrots in the preheated oven for about 20 minutes, until fork-tender.
- ❖ Toss the carrots with the fresh herbs and serve immediately. Enjoy

29) BEST BRAISED GREEN BEANS

Preparation Time: 15 minutes		Servings: 4

Ingredients:

- ✓ 4 tbsp olive oil
- ✓ 1 carrot, cut into matchsticks
- ✓ 1 ½ pounds green beans, trimmed
- ✓ 4 garlic cloves, peeled
- ✓ 1 bay laurel
- ✓ 1 ½ cups vegetable broth
- ✓ Sea salt and ground black pepper, to taste
- ✓ 1 lemon, cut into wedges

Directions:

- ❖ Heat the olive oil in a saucepan over medium flame. Once hot, fry the carrots and green beans for about 5 minutes, stirring periodically to promote even cooking.
- ❖ Add in the garlic and bay laurel and continue sautéing an additional 1 minute or until fragrant.
- ❖ Add in the broth, salt and black pepper and continue to simmer, covered, for about 9 minutes or until the green beans are tender.
- ❖ Taste, adjust the seasonings and serve with lemon wedges. Enjoy

30) BEST BRAISED KALE WITH SESAME SEEDS

Preparation Time: 10 minutes

Servings: 4

Ingredients:

- ✓ 1 cup vegetable broth
- ✓ 1 pound kale, cleaned, tough stems removed, torn into pieces
- ✓ 4 tbsp olive oil
- ✓ 6 garlic cloves, chopped
- ✓ 1 tsp paprika
- ✓ Kosher salt and ground black pepper, to taste
- ✓ 4 tbsp sesame seeds, lightly toasted

Directions:

- ❖ In a saucepan, bring the vegetable broth to a boil; add in the kale leaves and turn the heat to a simmer. Cook for about 5 minutes until kale has softened; reserve.
- ❖ Heat the oil in the same saucepan over medium heat. Once hot, sauté the garlic for about 30 seconds or until aromatic.
- ❖ Add in the reserved kale, paprika, salt and black pepper and let it cook for a few minutes more or until heated through.
- ❖ Garnish with lightly toasted sesame seeds and serve immediately. Enjoy

31) AUTUMN ROASTED VEGETABLES

Preparation Time: 45 minutes

Servings: 4

Ingredients:

- ✓ 1/2 pound carrots, slice into 1-inch chunks
- ✓ 1/2 pound parsnips, slice into 1-inch chunks
- ✓ 1/2 pound celery, slice into 1-inch chunks
- ✓ 1/2 pound sweet potatoes, slice into 1-inch chunks
- ✓ 1 large onion, slice into wedges
- ✓ 1/4 cup olive oil
- ✓ 1 tsp red pepper flakes
- ✓ 1 tsp dried basil
- ✓ 1 tsp dried oregano
- ✓ 1 tsp dried thyme
- ✓ Sea salt and freshly ground black pepper

Directions:

- ❖ Start by preheating your oven to 420 degrees F.
- ❖ Toss the vegetables with the olive oil and spices. Arrange them on a parchment-lined roasting pan.
- ❖ Roast for about 25 minutes. Stir the vegetables and continue to cook for 20 minutes more.
- ❖ Enjoy!

32) AUTHENTIC MOROCCAN TAGINE

Preparation Time: 30 minutes

Servings: 4

Ingredients:

- ✓ 3 tbsp olive oil
- ✓ 1 large shallot, chopped
- ✓ 1 tsp ginger, peeled and minced
- ✓ 4 garlic cloves, chopped
- ✓ 2 medium carrots, trimmed and chopped
- ✓ 2 medium parsnips, trimmed and chopped
- ✓ 2 medium sweet potatoes, peeled and cubed
- ✓ Sea salt and ground black pepper, to taste
- ✓ 1 tsp hot sauce
- ✓ 1 tsp fenugreek
- ✓ 1/2 tsp saffron
- ✓ 1/2 tsp caraway
- ✓ 2 large tomatoes, pureed
- ✓ 4 cups vegetable broth
- ✓ 1 lemon, cut into wedges

Directions:

- ❖ In a Dutch Oven, heat the olive oil over medium heat. Once hot, sauté the shallots for 4 to 5 minutes, until tender.
- ❖ Then, sauté the ginger and garlic for about 40 seconds or until aromatic.
- ❖ Add in the remaining ingredients, except for the lemon and bring to a boil. Immediately turn the heat to a simmer.
- ❖ Let it simmer for about 25 minutes or until the vegetables have softened. Serve with fresh lemon wedges and enjoy

33) CHINESE-STYLE CABBAGE STIR-FRY

Preparation Time: 10 minutes		Servings: 3

Ingredients:

- ✓ 3 tbsp sesame oil
- ✓ 1 pound Chinese cabbage, sliced
- ✓ 1/2 tsp Chinese five-spice powder
- ✓ Kosher salt, to taste
- ✓ 1/2 tsp Szechuan pepper
- ✓ 2 tbsp soy sauce
- ✓ 3 tbsp sesame seeds, lightly toasted

Directions:

- ❖ In a wok, heat the sesame oil until sizzling. Stir fry the cabbage for about 5 minutes.
- ❖ Stir in the spices and soy sauce and continue to cook, stirring frequently, for about 5 minutes more, until the cabbage is crisp-tender and aromatic.
- ❖ Sprinkle sesame seeds over the top and serve immediately

34) SPECIAL SAUTÉED CAULIFLOWER WITH SESAME SEEDS

Preparation Time: 15 minutes		Servings: 4

Ingredients:

- ✓ 1 cup vegetable broth
- ✓ 1 ½ pounds cauliflower florets
- ✓ 4 tbsp olive oil
- ✓ 2 scallion stalks, chopped
- ✓ 4 garlic cloves, minced
- ✓ Sea salt and freshly ground black pepper, to taste
- ✓ 2 tbsp sesame seeds, lightly toasted

Directions:

- ❖ In a large saucepan, bring the vegetable broth to a boil; then, add in the cauliflower and cook for about 6 minutes or until fork-tender; reserve.
- ❖ Then, heat the olive oil until sizzling; now, sauté the scallions and garlic for about 1 minute or until tender and aromatic.
- ❖ Add in the reserved cauliflower, followed by salt and black pepper; continue to simmer for about 5 minutes or until heated through
- ❖ Garnish with toasted sesame seeds and serve immediately. Enjoy

35) BEST SWEET MASHED CARROTS

Preparation Time: 25 minutes		Servings: 4

Ingredients:

- ✓ 1 ½ pounds carrots, trimmed
- ✓ 3 tbsp vegan butter
- ✓ 1 cup scallions, sliced
- ✓ 1 tbsp maple syrup
- ✓ 1/2 tsp garlic powder
- ✓ 1/2 tsp ground allspice
- ✓ Sea salt, to taste
- ✓ 1/2 cup soy sauce
- ✓ 2 tbsp fresh cilantro, chopped

Directions:

- ❖ Steam the carrots for about 15 minutes until they are very tender; drain well.
- ❖ In a sauté pan, melt the butter until sizzling. Now, turn the heat down to maintain an insistent sizzle.
- ❖ Now, cook the scallions until they've softened. Add in the maple syrup, garlic powder, ground allspice, salt and soy sauce for about 10 minutes or until they are caramelized.
- ❖ Add the caramelized scallions to your food processor; add in the carrots and puree the ingredients until everything is well blended.
- ❖ Serve garnished with the fresh cilantro. Enjoy

36) LOVELY SAUTÉED TURNIP GREENS

Preparation Time: 15 minutes | | **Servings:** 4

Ingredients:

- ✓ 2 tbsp olive oil
- ✓ 1 onion, sliced
- ✓ 2 garlic cloves, sliced
- ✓ 1 ½ pounds turnip greens cleaned and chopped
- ✓ 1/4 cup vegetable broth
- ✓ 1/4 cup dry white wine
- ✓ 1/2 tsp dried oregano
- ✓ 1 tsp dried parsley flakes
- ✓ Kosher salt and ground black pepper, to taste

Directions:

- ❖ In a sauté pan, heat the olive oil over a moderately high heat.
- ❖ Now, sauté the onion for 3 to 4 minutes or until tender and translucent. Add in the garlic and continue to cook for 30 seconds more or until aromatic.
- ❖ Stir in the turnip greens, broth, wine, oregano and parsley; continue sautéing an additional 6 minutes or until they have wilted completely.
- ❖ Season with salt and black pepper to taste and serve warm. Enjoy

37) ASIAN YUKON GOLD MASHED POTATOES

Preparation Time: 25 minutes | | **Servings:** 5

Ingredients:

- ✓ 2 pounds Yukon Gold potatoes, peeled and diced
- ✓ 1 clove garlic, pressed
- ✓ Sea salt and red pepper flakes, to taste
- ✓ 3 tbsp vegan butter
- ✓ 1/2 cup soy milk
- ✓ 2 tbsp scallions, sliced

Directions:

- ❖ Cover the potatoes with an inch or two of cold water. Cook the potatoes in gently boiling water for about 20 minutes.
- ❖ Then, puree the potatoes, along with the garlic, salt, red pepper, butter and milk, to your desired consistency.
- ❖ Serve garnished with fresh scallions. Enjoy

38) SUPER AROMATIC SAUTÉED SWISS CHARD

Preparation Time: 15 minutes | | **Servings:** 4

Ingredients:

- ✓ 2 tbsp vegan butter
- ✓ 1 onion, chopped
- ✓ 2 cloves garlic, sliced
- ✓ Sea salt and ground black pepper, to season
- ✓ 1 ½ pounds Swiss chard, torn into pieces, tough stalks removed
- ✓ 1 cup vegetable broth
- ✓ 1 bay leaf
- ✓ 1 thyme sprig
- ✓ 2 rosemary sprigs
- ✓ 1/2 tsp mustard seeds
- ✓ 1 tsp celery seeds

Directions:

- ❖ In a saucepan, melt the vegan butter over medium-high heat.
- ❖ Then, sauté the onion for about 3 minutes or until tender and translucent; sauté the garlic for about 1 minute until aromatic.
- ❖ Add in the remaining ingredients and turn the heat to a simmer; let it simmer, covered, for about 10 minutes or until everything is cooked through. Enjoy

39) TYPICAL SAUTÉED BELL PEPPERS

Preparation Time: 15 minutes | | **Servings:** 2

Ingredients:

- ✓ 3 tbsp olive oil
- ✓ 4 bell peppers, seeded and slice into strips
- ✓ 2 cloves garlic, minced
- ✓ Salt and freshly ground black pepper, to taste
- ✓ 1 tsp cayenne pepper
- ✓ 4 tbsp dry white wine
- ✓ 2 tbsp fresh cilantro, roughly chopped

Directions:

- ❖ In a saucepan, heat the oil over medium-high heat.
- ❖ Once hot, sauté the peppers for about 4 minutes or until tender and fragrant. Then, sauté the garlic for about 1 minute until aromatic.
- ❖ Add in the salt, black pepper and cayenne pepper; continue to sauté, adding the wine, for about 6 minutes more until tender and cooked through.
- ❖ Taste and adjust the seasonings. Top with fresh cilantro and serve. Enjoy

40) CLASSIC MASHED ROOT VEGETABLES

Preparation Time: 25 minutes | | **Servings:** 5

Ingredients:

- ✓ 1 pound russet potatoes, peeled and cut into chunks
- ✓ 1/2 pound parsnips, trimmed and diced
- ✓ 1/2 pound carrots, trimmed and diced
- ✓ 4 tbsp vegan butter
- ✓ 1 tsp dried oregano
- ✓ 1/2 tsp dried dill weed
- ✓ 1/2 tsp dried marjoram
- ✓ 1 tsp dried basil

Directions:

- ❖ Cover the vegetables with the water by 1 inch. Bring to a boil and cook for about 25 minutes until they've softened; drain.
- ❖ Mash the vegetables with the remaining ingredients, adding cooking liquid, as needed.
- ❖ Serve warm and enjoy

41) EASY ROASTED BUTTERNUT SQUASH

Preparation Time: 25 minutes | | **Servings:** 4

Ingredients:

- ✓ 4 tbsp olive oil
- ✓ 1/2 tsp ground cumin
- ✓ 1/2 tsp ground allspice
- ✓ 1 ½ pounds butternut squash, peeled, seeded and diced
- ✓ 1/4 cup dry white wine
- ✓ 2 tbsp dark soy sauce
- ✓ 1 tsp mustard seeds
- ✓ 1 tsp paprika
- ✓ Sea salt and ground black pepper, to taste

Directions:

- ❖ Start by preheating your oven to 420 degrees F. Toss the squash with the remaining ingredients.
- ❖ Roast the butternut squash for about 25 minutes or until tender and caramelized.
- ❖ Serve warm and enjoy

42) CLASSICAL SAUTÉED CREMINI MUSHROOMS

Preparation Time: 10 minutes		Servings: 4

Ingredients:

- ✓ 4 tbsp olive oil
- ✓ 4 tbsp shallots, chopped
- ✓ 2 cloves garlic, minced
- ✓ 1 ½ pounds Cremini mushrooms, sliced
- ✓ 1/4 cup dry white wine
- ✓ Sea salt and ground black pepper, to taste

Directions:

- ❖ In a sauté pan, heat the olive oil over a moderately high heat.
- ❖ Now, sauté the shallot for 3 to 4 minutes or until tender and translucent. Add in the garlic and continue to cook for 30 seconds more or until aromatic.
- ❖ Stir in the Cremini mushrooms, wine, salt and black pepper; continue sautéing an additional 6 minutes, until your mushrooms are lightly browned.
- ❖ Enjoy

43) EASY ROASTED ASPARAGUS WITH SESAME SEEDS

Preparation Time: 25 minutes		Servings: 4

Ingredients:

- ✓ 1 ½ pounds asparagus, trimmed
- ✓ 4 tbsp extra-virgin olive oil
- ✓ Sea salt and ground black pepper, to taste
- ✓ 1/2 tsp dried oregano
- ✓ 1/2 tsp dried basil
- ✓ 1 tsp red pepper flakes, crushed
- ✓ 4 tbsp sesame seeds
- ✓ 2 tbsp fresh chives, roughly chopped

Directions:

- ❖ Start by preheating the oven to 400 degrees F. Then, line a baking sheet with parchment paper.
- ❖ Toss the asparagus with the olive oil, salt, black pepper, oregano, basil and red pepper flakes. Now, arrange your asparagus in a single layer on the prepared baking sheet.
- ❖ Roast your asparagus for approximately 20 minutes.
- ❖ Sprinkle sesame seeds over your asparagus and continue to bake an additional 5 minutes or until the asparagus spears are crisp-tender and the sesame seeds are lightly toasted.
- ❖ Garnish with fresh chives and serve warm. Enjoy

44) SPECIAL GREEK-STYLE EGGPLANT SKILLET

Preparation Time: 15 minutes		Servings: 4

Ingredients:

- ✓ 4 tbsp olive oil
- ✓ 1 ½ pounds eggplant, peeled and sliced
- ✓ 1 tsp garlic, minced
- ✓ 1 tomato, crushed
- ✓ Sea salt and ground black pepper, to taste
- ✓ 1 tsp cayenne pepper
- ✓ 1/2 tsp dried oregano
- ✓ 1/4 tsp ground bay leaf
- ✓ 2 ounces Kalamata olives, pitted and sliced

Directions:

- ❖ Heat the oil in a sauté pan over medium-high flame.
- ❖ Then, sauté the eggplant for about 9 minutes or until just tender.
- ❖ Add in the remaining ingredients, cover and continue to cook for 2 to 3 minutes more or until thoroughly cooked. Serve warm

45) SIMPLE CAULIFLOWER RICE

Preparation Time: 10 minutes | | **Servings:** 5

Ingredients:

- ✓ 2 medium heads cauliflower, stems and leaves removed
- ✓ 4 tbsp extra-virgin olive oil
- ✓ 4 garlic cloves, pressed
- ✓ 1/2 tsp red pepper flakes, crushed
- ✓ Sea salt and ground black pepper, to taste
- ✓ 1/4 cup flat-leaf parsley, roughly chopped

Directions:

- ❖ Pulse the cauliflower in a food processor with the S-blade until they're broken into "rice".
- ❖ Heat the olive oil in a saucepan over medium-high heat. Once hot, cook the garlic until fragrant or about 1 minute.
- ❖ Add in the cauliflower rice, red pepper, salt and black pepper and continue sautéing for a further 7 to 8 minutes.
- ❖ Taste, adjust the seasonings and garnish with fresh parsley. Enjoy

46) SIMPLE GARLICKY KALE

Preparation Time: 10 minutes | | **Servings:** 4

Ingredients:

- ✓ 4 tbsp olive oil
- ✓ 4 cloves garlic, chopped
- ✓ 1 ½ pounds fresh kale, tough stems and ribs removed, torn into pieces
- ✓ 1 cup vegetable broth
- ✓ 1/2 tsp cumin seeds
- ✓ 1/2 tsp dried oregano
- ✓ 1/2 tsp paprika
- ✓ 1 tsp onion powder
- ✓ Sea salt and ground black pepper, to taste

Directions:

- ❖ In a saucepan, heat the olive oil over a moderately high heat. Now, sauté the garlic for about 1 minute or until aromatic.
- ❖ Add in the kale in batches, gradually adding the vegetable broth; stir to promote even cooking.
- ❖ Turn the heat to a simmer, add in the spices and let it cook for 5 to 6 minutes, until the kale leaves wilt.
- ❖ Serve warm and enjoy

47) ITALIAN ARTICHOKES BRAISED IN LEMON AND OLIVE OIL

Preparation Time: 35 minutes | | **Servings:** 4

Ingredients:

- ✓ 1 ½ cups water
- ✓ 2 lemons, freshly squeezed
- ✓ 2 pounds artichokes, trimmed, tough outer leaves and chokes removed
- ✓ 1 handful fresh Italian parsley
- ✓ 2 thyme sprigs
- ✓ 2 rosemary sprigs
- ✓ 2 bay leaves
- ✓ 2 garlic cloves, chopped
- ✓ 1/3 cup olive oil
- ✓ Sea salt and ground black pepper, to taste
- ✓ 1/2 tsp red pepper flakes

Directions:

- ❖ Fill a bowl with water and add in the lemon juice. Place the cleaned artichokes in the bowl, keeping them completely submerged.
- ❖ In another small bowl, thoroughly combine the herbs and garlic. Rub your artichokes with the herb mixture.
- ❖ Pour the lemon water and olive oil in a saucepan; add the artichokes to the saucepan. Turn the heat to a simmer and continue to cook, covered, for about 30 minutes until the artichokes are crisp-tender.
- ❖ To serve, drizzle the artichokes with cooking juices, season them with the salt, black pepper and red pepper flakes. Enjoy

48) MEDITERRANEAN ROSEMARY AND GARLIC ROASTED CARROTS

Preparation Time: 25 minutes | | **Servings:** 4

Ingredients:

- ✓ 2 pounds carrots, trimmed and halved lengthwise
- ✓ 4 tbsp olive oil
- ✓ 2 tbsp champagne vinegar
- ✓ 4 cloves garlic, minced
- ✓ 2 sprigs rosemary, chopped
- ✓ Sea salt and ground black pepper, to taste
- ✓ 4 tbsp pine nuts, chopped

Directions:

- ❖ Begin by preheating your oven to 400 degrees F.
- ❖ Toss the carrots with the olive oil, vinegar, garlic, rosemary, salt and black pepper. Arrange them in a single layer on a parchment-lined roasting sheet.
- ❖ Roast the carrots in the preheated oven for about 20 minutes, until fork-tender.
- ❖ Garnish the carrots with the pine nuts and serve immediately. Enjoy

49) EASY MEDITERRANEAN-STYLE GREEN BEANS

Preparation Time: 20 minutes | | **Servings:** 4

Ingredients:

- ✓ 2 tbsp olive oil
- ✓ 1 red bell pepper, seeded and diced
- ✓ 1 ½ pounds green beans
- ✓ 4 garlic cloves, minced
- ✓ 1/2 tsp mustard seeds
- ✓ 1/2 tsp fennel seeds
- ✓ 1 tsp dried dill weed
- ✓ 2 tomatoes, pureed
- ✓ 1 cup cream of celery soup
- ✓ 1 tsp Italian herb mix
- ✓ 1 tsp cayenne pepper
- ✓ Salt and freshly ground black pepper

Directions:

- ❖ Heat the olive oil in a saucepan over medium flame. Once hot, fry the peppers and green beans for about 5 minutes, stirring periodically to promote even cooking.
- ❖ Add in the garlic, mustard seeds, fennel seeds and dill and continue sautéing an additional 1 minute or until fragrant.
- ❖ Add in the pureed tomatoes, cream of celery soup, Italian herb mix, cayenne pepper, salt and black pepper. Continue to simmer, covered, for about 9 minutes or until the green beans are tender.
- ❖ Taste, adjust the seasonings and serve warm. Enjoy

50) SIMPLE ROASTED GARDEN VEGETABLES

Preparation Time: 45 minutes | | **Servings:** 4

Ingredients:

- ✓ 1 pound butternut squash, peeled and cut into 1-inch pieces
- ✓ 4 sweet potatoes, peeled and cut into 1-inch pieces
- ✓ 1/2 cup carrots, peeled and cut into 1-inch pieces
- ✓ 2 medium onions, cut into wedges
- ✓ 4 tbsp olive oil
- ✓ 1 tsp granulated garlic
- ✓ 1 tsp paprika
- ✓ 1 tsp dried rosemary
- ✓ 1 tsp mustard seeds
- ✓ Kosher salt and freshly ground black pepper, to taste

Directions:

- ❖ Start by preheating your oven to 420 degrees F.
- ❖ Toss the vegetables with the olive oil and spices. Arrange them on a parchment-lined roasting pan.
- ❖ Roast for about 25 minutes. Stir the vegetables and continue to cook for 20 minutes more.
- ❖ Enjoy

51) QUICK ROASTED KOHLRABI

Preparation Time: 30 minutes		Servings: 4

Ingredients:

- ✓ 1 pound kohlrabi bulbs, peeled and sliced
- ✓ 4 tbsp olive oil
- ✓ 1/2 tsp mustard seeds
- ✓ 1 tsp celery seeds
- ✓ 1 tsp dried marjoram
- ✓ 1 tsp granulated garlic, minced
- ✓ Sea salt and ground black pepper, to taste
- ✓ 2 tbsp nutritional yeast

Directions:

- ❖ Start by preheating your oven to 450 degrees F.
- ❖ Toss the kohlrabi with the olive oil and spices until well coated. Arrange the kohlrabi in a single layer on a parchment-lined roasting pan.
- ❖ Bake the kohlrabi in the preheated oven for about 15 minutes; stir them and continue to cook an additional 15 minutes.
- ❖ Sprinkle nutritional yeast over the warm kohlrabi and serve immediately. Enjoy

52) SPECIAL CAULIFLOWER WITH TAHINI SAUCE

Preparation Time: 10 minutes		Servings: 4

Ingredients:

- ✓ 1 cup water
- ✓ 2 pounds cauliflower florets
- ✓ Sea salt and ground black pepper, to taste
- ✓ 3 tbsp soy sauce
- ✓ 5 tbsp tahini
- ✓ 2 cloves garlic, minced
- ✓ 2 tbsp lemon juice

Directions:

- ❖ In a large saucepan, bring the water to a boil; then, add in the cauliflower and cook for about 6 minutes or until fork-tender; drain, season with salt and pepper and reserve.
- ❖ In a mixing bowl, thoroughly combine the soy sauce, tahini, garlic and lemon juice. Spoon the sauce over the cauliflower florets and serve.
- ❖ Enjoy

53) ITALIAN-STYLE HERB CAULIFLOWER MASH

Preparation Time: 25 minutes		Servings: 4

Ingredients:

- ✓ 1 ½ pounds cauliflower florets
- ✓ 4 tbsp vegan butter
- ✓ 4 cloves garlic, sliced
- ✓ Sea salt and ground black pepper, to taste
- ✓ 1/4 cup plain oat milk, unsweetened
- ✓ 2 tbsp fresh parsley, roughly chopped

Directions:

- ❖ Steam the cauliflower florets for about 20 minutes; set it aside to cool.
- ❖ In a saucepan, melt the vegan butter over a moderately high heat; now, sauté the garlic for about 1 minute or until aromatic.
- ❖ Add the cauliflower florets to your food processor followed by the sautéed garlic, salt, black pepper and oat milk. Puree until everything is well incorporated.
- ❖ Garnish with fresh parsley leaves and serve hot. Enjoy

54) BEST GARLIC AND HERB MUSHROOM SKILLET

Preparation Time: 10 minutes		Servings: 4

Ingredients:

- ✓ 4 tbsp vegan butter
- ✓ 1 ½ pounds oyster mushrooms halved
- ✓ 3 cloves garlic, minced
- ✓ 1 tsp dried oregano
- ✓ 1 tsp dried rosemary
- ✓ 1 tsp dried parsley flakes
- ✓ 1 tsp dried marjoram
- ✓ 1/2 cup dry white wine
- ✓ Kosher salt and ground black pepper, to taste

Directions:

- ❖ In a sauté pan, heat the olive oil over a moderately high heat.
- ❖ Now, sauté the mushrooms for 3 minutes or until they release the liquid. Add in the garlic and continue to cook for 30 seconds more or until aromatic.
- ❖ Stir in the spices and continue sautéing an additional 6 minutes, until your mushrooms are lightly browned.
- ❖ Enjoy

Chapter 3. DINNER

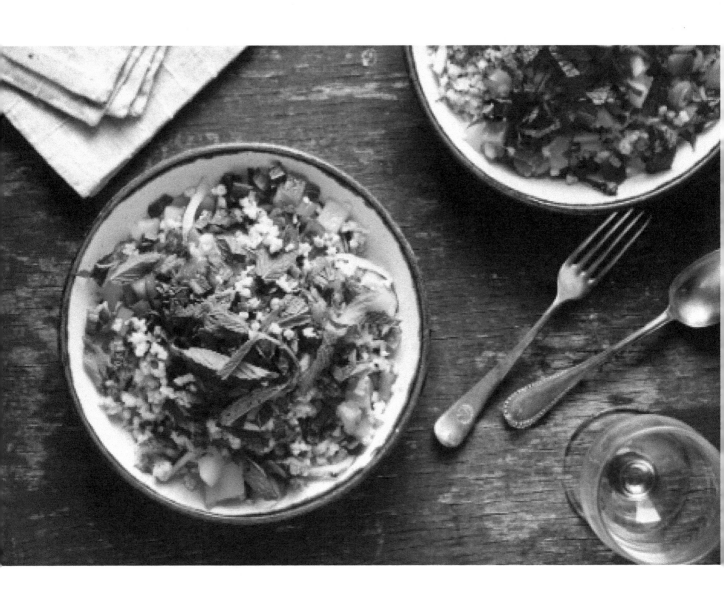

55) SIMPLE PAN-FRIED ASPARAGUS

Preparation Time: 10 minutes | | **Servings:** 4

Ingredients:

- ✓ 4 tbsp vegan butter
- ✓ 1 ½ pounds asparagus spears, trimmed
- ✓ 1/2 tsp cumin seeds, ground
- ✓ 1/4 tsp bay leaf, ground
- ✓ Sea salt and ground black pepper, to taste
- ✓ 1 tsp fresh lime juice

Directions:

- ❖ Melt the vegan butter in a saucepan over medium-high heat.
- ❖ Sauté the asparagus for about 3 to 4 minutes, stirring periodically to promote even cooking.
- ❖ Add in the cumin seeds, bay leaf, salt and black pepper and continue to cook the asparagus for 2 minutes more until crisp-tender.
- ❖ Drizzle lime juice over the asparagus and serve warm. Enjoy

56) EASY GINGERY CARROT MASH

Preparation Time: 25 minutes | | **Servings:** 4

Ingredients:

- ✓ 2 pounds carrots, cut into rounds
- ✓ 2 tbsp olive oil
- ✓ 1 tsp ground cumin
- ✓ Salt ground black pepper, to taste
- ✓ 1/2 tsp cayenne pepper
- ✓ 1/2 tsp ginger, peeled and minced
- ✓ 1/2 cup whole milk

Directions:

- ❖ Begin by preheating your oven to 400 degrees F.
- ❖ Toss the carrots with the olive oil, cumin, salt, black pepper and cayenne pepper. Arrange them in a single layer on a parchment-lined roasting sheet.
- ❖ Roast the carrots in the preheated oven for about 20 minutes, until crisp-tender.
- ❖ Add the roasted carrots, ginger and milk to your food processor; puree the ingredients until everything is well blended.
- ❖ Enjoy

57) ONLY MEDITERRANEAN-STYLE ROASTED ARTICHOKES

Preparation Time: 50 minutes | | **Servings:** 4

Ingredients:

- ✓ 4 artichokes, trimmed, tough outer leaves and chokes removed, halved
- ✓ 2 lemons, freshly squeezed
- ✓ 4 tbsp extra-virgin olive oil
- ✓ 4 cloves garlic, chopped
- ✓ 1 tsp fresh rosemary
- ✓ 1 tsp fresh basil
- ✓ 1 tsp fresh parsley
- ✓ 1 tsp fresh oregano
- ✓ Flaky sea salt and ground black pepper, to taste
- ✓ 1 tsp red pepper flakes
- ✓ 1 tsp paprika

Directions:

- ❖ Start by preheating your oven to 395 degrees F. Rub the lemon juice all over the entire surface of your artichokes.
- ❖ In a small mixing bowl, thoroughly combine the garlic with herbs and spices
- ❖ Place the artichoke halves in a parchment-lined baking dish, cut-side-up. Brush the artichokes evenly with the olive oil. Fill the cavities with the garlic/herb mixture.
- ❖ Bake for about 20 minutes. Now, cover them with aluminum foil and bake for a further 30 minutes. Serve warm and enjoy

58) ASIAN THAI-STYLE BRAISED KALE

Preparation Time: 10 minutes | | **Servings: 4**

Ingredients:

- ✓ 1 cup water
- ✓ 1 ½ pounds kale, tough stems and ribs removed, torn into pieces
- ✓ 2 tbsp sesame oil
- ✓ 1 tsp fresh garlic, pressed
- ✓ 1 tsp ginger, peeled and minced
- ✓ 1 Thai chili, chopped
- ✓ 1/2 tsp turmeric powder
- ✓ 1/2 cup coconut milk
- ✓ Kosher salt and ground black pepper, to taste

Directions:

- ❖ In a large saucepan, bring the water to a rapid boil. Add in the kale and let it cook until bright, about 3 minutes. Drain, rinse and squeeze dry.
- ❖ Wipe the saucepan with paper towels and preheat the sesame oil over a moderate heat. Once hot, cook the garlic, ginger and chili for approximately 1 minute or so, until fragrant.
- ❖ Add in the kale and turmeric powder and continue to cook for a further 1 minute or until heated through.
- ❖ Gradually pour in the coconut milk, salt and black pepper; continue to simmer until the liquid has thickened. Taste, adjust the seasonings and serve hot. Enjoy

59) SPECIAL SILKY KOHLRABI PUREE

Preparation Time: 30 minutes | | **Servings: 4**

Ingredients:

- ✓ 1 ½ pounds kohlrabi, peeled and cut into pieces
- ✓ 4 tbsp vegan butter
- ✓ Sea salt and freshly ground black pepper, to taste
- ✓ 1/2 tsp cumin seeds
- ✓ 1/2 tsp coriander seeds
- ✓ 1/2 cup soy milk
- ✓ 1 tsp fresh dill
- ✓ 1 tsp fresh parsley

Directions:

- ❖ Cook the kohlrabi in boiling salted water until soft, about 30 minutes; drain.
- ❖ Puree the kohlrabi with the vegan butter, salt, black pepper, cumin seeds and coriander seeds.
- ❖ Puree the ingredients with an immersion blender, gradually adding the milk. Top with fresh dill and parsley. Enjoy

60) TASTY CREAMY SAUTÉED SPINACH

Preparation Time: 15 minutes | | **Servings: 4**

Ingredients:

- ✓ 2 tbsp vegan butter
- ✓ 1 onion, chopped
- ✓ 1 tsp garlic, minced
- ✓ 1 ½ cups vegetable broth
- ✓ 2 pounds spinach, torn into pieces
- ✓ Sea salt and ground black pepper, to taste
- ✓ 1/4 tsp dried dill
- ✓ 1/4 tsp mustard seeds
- ✓ 1/2 tsp celery seeds
- ✓ 1 tsp cayenne pepper
- ✓ 1/2 cup oat milk

Directions:

- ❖ In a saucepan, melt the vegan butter over medium-high heat.
- ❖ Then, sauté the onion for about 3 minutes or until tender and translucent. Then, sauté the garlic for about 1 minute until aromatic.
- ❖ Add in the broth and spinach and bring to a boil.
- ❖ Turn the heat to a simmer. Add in the spices and continue to cook for 5 minutes longer.
- ❖ Add in the milk and continue to cook for 5 minutes more. Enjoy

61) DELICIOUS SWEET AND SPICY BRUSSEL SPROUT STIR-FRY

Preparation Time: 15 minutes

Servings: 4

Ingredients:

- ✓ 4 oz plant butter + more to taste
- ✓ 4 shallots, chopped
- ✓ 1 tbsp apple cider vinegar
- ✓ Salt and black pepper to taste
- ✓ 1 lb Brussels sprouts
- ✓ Hot chili sauce

Directions:

- ❖ Put the plant butter in a saucepan and melt over medium heat. Pour in the shallots and sauté for 2 minutes, to caramelize and slightly soften. Add the apple cider vinegar, salt, and black pepper. Stir and reduce the heat to cook the shallots further with continuous stirring, about 5 minutes. Transfer to a plate after.
- ❖ Trim the Brussel sprouts and cut in halves. Leave the small ones as wholes. Pour the Brussel sprouts into the saucepan and stir-fry with more plant butter until softened but al dente. Season with salt and black pepper, stir in the onions and hot chili sauce, and heat for a few seconds. Serve immediately

62) MEXICAN BLACK BEAN BURGERS WITH BBQ SAUCE

Preparation Time: 20 minutes

Servings: 4

Ingredients:

- ✓ 3 (15 oz) cans black beans, drained
- ✓ 2 tbsp whole-wheat flour
- ✓ 2 tbsp quick-cooking oats
- ✓ ¼ cup chopped fresh basil
- ✓ 2 tbsp pure barbecue sauce
- ✓ 1 garlic clove, minced
- ✓ Salt and black pepper to taste
- ✓ 4 whole-grain hamburger buns, split
- ✓ For topping:
- ✓ Red onion slices
- ✓ Tomato slices
- ✓ Fresh basil leaves
- ✓ Additional barbecue sauce

Directions:

- ❖ In a medium bowl, mash the black beans and mix in the flour, oats, basil, barbecue sauce, garlic salt, and black pepper until well combined. Mold 4 patties out of the mixture and set aside.
- ❖ Heat a grill pan to medium heat and lightly grease with cooking spray. Cook the bean patties on both sides until light brown and cooked through, 10 minutes. Place the patties between the burger buns and top with the onions, tomatoes, basil, and some barbecue sauce. Serve warm

63) LOVELY CREAMY BRUSSELS SPROUTS BAKE

Preparation Time: 26 minutes

Servings: 4

Ingredients:

- ✓ 3 tbsp plant butter
- ✓ 1 cup tempeh, cut into 1-inch cubes
- ✓ 1 ½ lb halved Brussels sprouts
- ✓ 5 garlic cloves, minced
- ✓ 1 ¼ cups coconut cream
- ✓ 10 oz grated plant-based mozzarella
- ✓ ¼ cup grated plant-based Parmesan
- ✓ Salt and black pepper to taste

Directions:

- ❖ Preheat oven to 400 F.
- ❖ Melt the plant butter in a large skillet over medium heat and fry the tempeh cubes until browned on both sides, about 6 minutes. Remove onto a plate and set aside. Pour the Brussels sprouts and garlic into the skillet and sauté until fragrant.
- ❖ Mix in coconut cream and simmer for 4 minutes. Add tempeh cubes and combine well. Pour the sauté into a baking dish, sprinkle with plant-based mozzarella cheese, and plant-based Parmesan cheese. Bake for 10 minutes or until golden brown on top. Serve with tomato salad

64) GENOVESE BASIL PESTO SEITAN PANINI

Preparation Time: 15 minutes+ cooling time		Servings: 4

Ingredients:

- For the seitan:
- 2/3 cup basil pesto
- ½ lemon, juiced
- 1 garlic clove, minced
- 1/8 tsp salt
- 1 cup chopped seitan
- For the panini:
- 3 tbsp basil pesto
- 8 thick slices whole-wheat ciabatta
- Olive oil for brushing
- 8 slices plant-based mozzarella
- 1 yellow bell pepper, chopped
- ¼ cup grated plant Parmesan cheese

Directions:

- In a medium bowl, mix the pesto, lemon juice, garlic, and salt. Add the seitan and coat well with the marinade. Cover with plastic wrap and marinate in the refrigerator for 30 minutes.
- Preheat a large skillet over medium heat and remove the seitan from the fridge. Cook the seitan in the skillet until brown and cooked through, 2-3 minutes. Turn the heat off.
- Preheat a panini press to medium heat. In a small bowl, mix the pesto in the inner parts of two slices of bread. On the outer parts, apply some olive oil and place a slice with (the olive oil side down) in the press. Lay 2 slices of plant-based mozzarella cheese on the bread, spoon some seitan on top. Sprinkle with some bell pepper and some plant-based Parmesan cheese. Cover with another bread slice.
- Close the press and grill the bread for 1 to 2 minutes. Flip the bread, and grill further for 1 minute or until the cheese melts and golden brown on both sides. Serve warm

65) ENGLISH SWEET OATMEAL "GRITS"

Preparation Time: 20 minutes		Servings: 4

Ingredients:

- 1 ½ cups steel-cut oats, soaked overnight
- 1 cup almond milk
- 2 cups water
- A pinch of grated nutmeg
- A pinch of ground cloves
- A pinch of sea salt
- 4 tbsp almonds, slivered
- 6 dates, pitted and chopped
- 6 prunes, chopped

Directions:

- In a deep saucepan, bring the steel cut oats, almond milk and water to a boil.
- Add in the nutmeg, cloves and salt. Immediately turn the heat to a simmer, cover and continue to cook for about 15 minutes or until they've softened.
- Then, spoon the grits into four serving bowls; top them with the almonds, dates and prunes.
- Enjoy!

66) SPECIAL FREEKEH BOWL WITH DRIED FIGS

Preparation Time: 35 minutes		Servings: 2

Ingredients:

- 1/2 cup freekeh, soaked for 30 minutes, drained
- 1 1/3 cups almond milk
- 1/4 tsp sea salt
- 1/4 tsp ground cloves
- 1/4 tsp ground cinnamon
- 4 tbsp agave syrup
- 2 ounces dried figs, chopped

Directions:

- Place the freekeh, milk, sea salt, ground cloves and cinnamon in a saucepan. Bring to a boil over medium-high heat.
- Immediately turn the heat to a simmer for 30 to 35 minutes, stirring occasionally to promote even cooking.
- Stir in the agave syrup and figs. Ladle the porridge into individual bowls and serve. Enjoy

67) EASY CORNMEAL PORRIDGE WITH MAPLE SYRUP

Preparation Time: 20 minutes | | **Servings:** 4

Ingredients:

- ✓ 2 cups water
- ✓ 2 cups almond milk
- ✓ 1 cinnamon stick
- ✓ 1 vanilla bean
- ✓ 1 cup yellow cornmeal
- ✓ 1/2 cup maple syrup

Directions:

- ❖ In a saucepan, bring the water and almond milk to a boil. Add in the cinnamon stick and vanilla bean.
- ❖ Gradually add in the cornmeal, stirring continuously; turn the heat to a simmer. Let it simmer for about 15 minutes.
- ❖ Drizzle the maple syrup over the porridge and serve warm. Enjoy

68) EVERYDAY MEDITERRANEAN-STYLE RICE

Preparation Time: 20 minutes | | **Servings:** 4

Ingredients:

- ✓ 3 tbsp vegan butter, at room temperature
- ✓ 4 tbsp scallions, chopped
- ✓ 2 cloves garlic, minced
- ✓ 1 bay leaf
- ✓ 1 thyme sprig, chopped
- ✓ 1 rosemary sprig, chopped
- ✓ 1 ½ cups white rice
- ✓ 2 cups vegetable broth
- ✓ 1 large tomato, pureed
- ✓ Sea salt and ground black pepper, to taste
- ✓ 2 ounces Kalamata olives, pitted and sliced

Directions:

- ❖ In a saucepan, melt the vegan butter over a moderately high flame. Cook the scallions for about 2 minutes or until tender.
- ❖ Add in the garlic, bay leaf, thyme and rosemary and continue to sauté for about 1 minute or until aromatic.
- ❖ Add in the rice, broth and pureed tomato. Bring to a boil; immediately turn the heat to a gentle simmer.
- ❖ Cook for about 15 minutes or until all the liquid has absorbed. Fluff the rice with a fork, season with salt and pepper and garnish with olives; serve immediately. Enjoy

69) MOROCCAN BULGUR PANCAKES WITH A TWIST

Preparation Time: 50 minutes | | **Servings:** 4

Ingredients:

- ✓ 1/2 cup bulgur wheat flour
- ✓ 1/2 cup almond flour
- ✓ 1 tsp baking soda
- ✓ 1/2 tsp fine sea salt
- ✓ 1 cup full-fat coconut milk
- ✓ 1/2 tsp ground cinnamon
- ✓ 1/4 tsp ground cloves
- ✓ 4 tbsp coconut oil
- ✓ 1/2 cup maple syrup
- ✓ 1 large-sized banana, sliced

Directions:

- ❖ In a mixing bowl, thoroughly combine the flour, baking soda, salt, coconut milk, cinnamon and ground cloves; let it stand for 30 minutes to soak well.
- ❖ Heat a small amount of the coconut oil in a frying pan.
- ❖ Fry the pancakes until the surface is golden brown. Garnish with maple syrup and banana. Enjoy

70) SIMPLE CHOCOLATE RYE PORRIDGE

Preparation Time: 10 minutes | | **Servings:** 4

Ingredients:

- ✓ 2 cups rye flakes
- ✓ 2 ½ cups almond milk
- ✓ 2 ounces dried prunes, chopped
- ✓ 2 ounces dark chocolate chunks

Directions:

- ❖ Add the rye flakes and almond milk to a deep saucepan; bring to a boil over medium-high. Turn the heat to a simmer and let it cook for 5 to 6 minutes.
- ❖ Remove from the heat. Fold in the chopped prunes and chocolate chunks, gently stir to combine.
- ❖ Ladle into serving bowls and serve warm.
- ❖ Enjoy

71) CLASSIC AFRICAN MIELIE-MEAL

Preparation Time: 15 minutes		Servings: 4

Ingredients:

- ✓ 3 cups water
- ✓ 1 cup coconut milk
- ✓ 1 cup maize meal
- ✓ 1/3 tsp kosher salt
- ✓ 1/4 tsp grated nutmeg
- ✓ 1/4 tsp ground cloves
- ✓ 4 tbsp maple syrup

Directions:

- ❖ In a saucepan, bring the water and milk to a boil; then, gradually add in the maize meal and turn the heat to a simmer.
- ❖ Add in the salt, nutmeg and cloves. Let it cook for 10 minutes.
- ❖ Add in the maple syrup and gently stir to combine. Enjoy

72) SPECIAL TEFF PORRIDGE WITH DRIED FIGS

Preparation Time: 25 minutes		Servings: 4

Ingredients:

- ✓ 1 cup whole-grain teff
- ✓ 1 cup water
- ✓ 2 cups coconut milk
- ✓ 2 tbsp coconut oil
- ✓ 1/2 tsp ground cardamom
- ✓ 1/4 tsp ground cinnamon
- ✓ 4 tbsp agave syrup
- ✓ 7-8 dried figs, chopped

Directions:

- ❖ Bring the whole-grain teff, water and coconut milk to a boil.
- ❖ Turn the heat to a simmer and add in the coconut oil, cardamom and cinnamon.
- ❖ Let it cook for 20 minutes or until the grain has softened and the porridge has thickened. Stir in the agave syrup and stir to combine well.
- ❖ Top each serving bowl with chopped figs and serve warm. Enjoy

73) TASTY DECADENT BREAD PUDDING WITH APRICOTS

Preparation Time: 1 hour		Servings: 4

Ingredients:

- ✓ 4 cups day-old ciabatta bread, cubed
- ✓ 4 tbsp coconut oil, melted
- ✓ 2 cups coconut milk
- ✓ 1/2 cup coconut sugar
- ✓ 4 tbsp applesauce
- ✓ 1/4 tsp ground cloves
- ✓ 1/2 tsp ground cinnamon
- ✓ 1 tsp vanilla extract
- ✓ 1/3 cup dried apricots, diced

Directions:

- ❖ Start by preheating your oven to 360 degrees F. Lightly oil a casserole dish with a nonstick cooking spray.
- ❖ Place the cubed bread in the prepared casserole dish.
- ❖ In a mixing bowl, thoroughly combine the coconut oil, milk, coconut sugar, applesauce, ground cloves, ground cinnamon and vanilla. Pour the custard evenly over the bread cubes; fold in the apricots.
- ❖ Press with a wide spatula and let it soak for about 15 minutes.
- ❖ Bake in the preheated oven for about 45 minutes or until the top is golden and set. Enjoy

74) TRADITIONAL CHIPOTLE CILANTRO RICE

Preparation Time: 25 minutes | | **Servings:** 4

Ingredients:

- ✓ 4 tbsp olive oil
- ✓ 1 chipotle pepper, seeded and chopped
- ✓ 1 cup jasmine rice
- ✓ 1 ½ cups vegetable broth
- ✓ 1/4 cup fresh cilantro, chopped
- ✓ Sea salt and cayenne pepper, to taste

Directions:

- ❖ In a saucepan, heat the olive oil over a moderately high flame. Add in the pepper and rice and cook for about 3 minutes or until aromatic.
- ❖ Pour the vegetable broth into the saucepan and bring to a boil; immediately turn the heat to a gentle simmer.
- ❖ Cook for about 18 minutes or until all the liquid has absorbed. Fluff the rice with a fork, add in the cilantro, salt and cayenne pepper; stir to combine well. Enjoy

75) ENGLISH OAT PORRIDGE WITH ALMONDS

Preparation Time: 20 minutes | | **Servings:** 2

Ingredients:

- ✓ 1 cup water
- ✓ 2 cups almond milk, divided
- ✓ 1 cup rolled oats
- ✓ 2 tbsp coconut sugar
- ✓ 1/2 vanilla essence
- ✓ 1/4 tsp cardamom
- ✓ 1/2 cup almonds, chopped
- ✓ 1 banana, sliced

Directions:

- ❖ In a deep saucepan, bring the water and milk to a rapid boil. Add in the oats, cover the saucepan and turn the heat to medium.
- ❖ Add in the coconut sugar, vanilla and cardamom. Continue to cook for about 12 minutes, stirring periodically.
- ❖ Spoon the mixture into serving bowls; top with almonds and banana. Enjoy

76) MEXICAN-STYLE JALAPEÑO QUINOA BOWL WITH LIMA BEANS

Preparation Time: 30 minutes | | **Servings:** 4

Ingredients:

- ✓ 1 tbsp olive oil
- ✓ 1 lb extra firm tofu, cubed
- ✓ Salt and black pepper to taste
- ✓ 1 medium yellow onion, finely diced
- ✓ ½ cup cauliflower florets
- ✓ 1 jalapeño pepper, minced
- ✓ 2 garlic cloves, minced
- ✓ 1 tbsp red chili powder
- ✓ 1 tsp cumin powder
- ✓ 1 (8 oz) can sweet corn kernels
- ✓ 1 (8 oz) can lima beans, rinsed
- ✓ 1 cup quick-cooking quinoa
- ✓ 1 (14 oz) can diced tomatoes
- ✓ 2 ½ cups vegetable broth
- ✓ 1 cup grated plant-based cheddar
- ✓ 2 tbsp chopped fresh cilantro
- ✓ 2 limes, cut into wedges
- ✓ 1 avocado, pitted, sliced, and peeled

Directions:

- ❖ Heat olive oil in a pot and cook the tofu until golden brown, 5 minutes. Season with salt, pepper, and mix in onion, cauliflower, and jalapeño pepper. Cook until the vegetables soften, 3 minutes.
- ❖ Stir in garlic, chili powder, and cumin powder; cook for 1 minute. Mix in sweet corn kernels, lima beans, quinoa, tomatoes, and vegetable broth. Simmer until the quinoa absorbs all the liquid, 10 minutes. Fluff quinoa. Top with the plant-based cheddar cheese, cilantro, lime wedges, and avocado. Serve

Chapter 4. DESSERTS

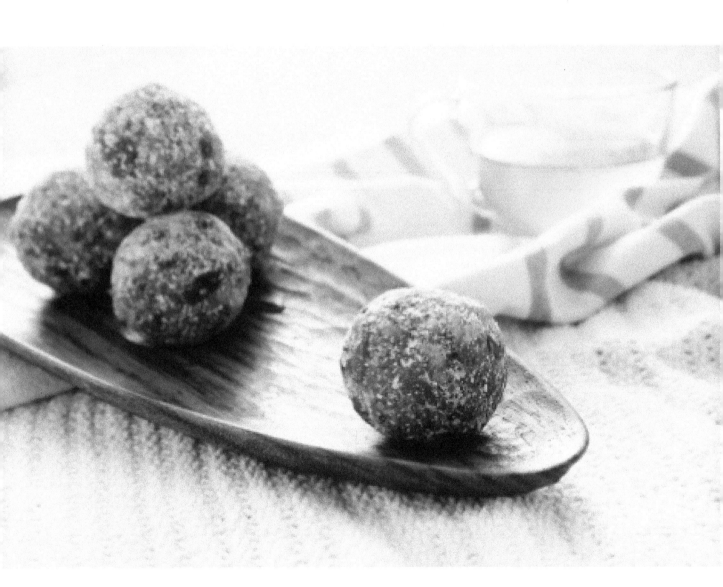

77) SOUTHERN AMERICAN APPLE COBBLER WITH RASPBERRIES

Preparation Time: 50 minutes		**Servings:** 4

Ingredients:

- ✓ 3 apples, chopped
- ✓ 2 tbsp pure date sugar
- ✓ 1 cup fresh raspberries
- ✓ 2 tbsp unsalted plant butter
- ✓ ½ cup whole-wheat flour
- ✓ 1 cup toasted rolled oats
- ✓ 2 tbsp pure date sugar
- ✓ 1 tsp cinnamon powder

Directions:

- ❖ Preheat the oven to 350 F and grease a baking dish with some plant butter.
- ❖ Add apples, date sugar, and 3 tbsp of water to a pot. Cook over low heat until the date sugar melts and then mix in the raspberries. Cook until the fruits soften, 10 minutes. Pour and spread the fruit mixture into the baking dish and set aside.
- ❖ In a blender, add the plant butter, flour, oats, date sugar, and cinnamon powder. Pulse a few times until crumbly. Spoon and spread the mixture on the fruit mix until evenly layered. Bake in the oven for 25 to 30 minutes or until golden brown on top. Remove the dessert, allow cooling for 2 minutes, and serve

78) SWEET CHOCOLATE PEPPERMINT MOUSSE

Preparation Time: 10 minutes + chilling time		**Servings:** 4

Ingredients:

- ✓ ¼ cup Swerve sugar, divided
- ✓ 4 oz cashew cream cheese, softened
- ✓ 3 tbsp cocoa powder
- ✓ ¾ tsp peppermint extract
- ✓ ½ tsp vanilla extract
- ✓ 1/3 cup coconut cream

Directions:

- ❖ Put 2 tbsp of Swerve sugar, cashew cream cheese, and cocoa powder in a blender. Add the peppermint extract, ¼ cup warm water, and process until smooth. In a bowl, whip vanilla extract, coconut cream, and the remaining Swerve sugar using a whisk. Fetch out 5-6 tbsp for garnishing. Fold in the cocoa mixture until thoroughly combined. Spoon the mousse into serving cups and chill in the fridge for 30 minutes. Garnish with the reserved whipped cream and serve

79) TASTY RASPBERRIES TURMERIC PANNA COTTA

Preparation Time: 10 minutes + chilling time		**Servings:** 6

Ingredients:

- ✓ ½ tbsp powdered vegetarian gelatin
- ✓ 2 cups coconut cream
- ✓ ¼ tsp vanilla extract
- ✓ 1 pinch turmeric powder
- ✓ 1 tbsp erythritol
- ✓ 1 tbsp chopped toasted pecans
- ✓ 12 fresh raspberries

Directions:

- ❖ Mix gelatin and ½ tsp water and allow sitting to dissolve. Pour coconut cream, vanilla extract, turmeric, and erythritol into a saucepan and bring to a boil over medium heat, then simmer for 2 minutes. Turn the heat off. Stir in the gelatin until dissolved. Pour the mixture into 6 glasses, cover with plastic wrap, and refrigerate for 2 hours or more. Top with the pecans and raspberries and serve

80) SPRING BANANA PUDDING

Preparation Time: 25 minutes + cooling time		Servings: 4

Ingredients:

- ✓ 1 cup unsweetened almond milk
- ✓ 2 cups cashew cream
- ✓ ¾ cup + 1 tbsp pure date sugar
- ✓ ¼ tsp salt
- ✓ 3 tbsp corn-starch
- ✓ 2 tbsp plant butter, cut into 4 pieces
- ✓ 1 tsp vanilla extract
- ✓ 2 banana, sliced

Directions:

❖ In a medium pot, mix almond milk, cashew cream, date sugar, and salt. Cook over medium heat until slightly thickened, 10-15 minutes. Stir in the corn-starch, plant butter, vanilla extract, and banana extract. Cook further for 1 to 2 minutes or until the pudding thickens. Dish the pudding into 4 serving bowls and chill in the refrigerator for at least 1 hour. To serve, top with the bananas and enjoy

81) EVERYDAY BAKED APPLES FILLED WITH NUTS

Preparation Time: 35 minutes + cooling time		Servings: 4

Ingredients:

- ✓ 4 gala apples
- ✓ 3 tbsp pure maple syrup
- ✓ 4 tbsp almond flour
- ✓ 6 tbsp pure date sugar
- ✓ 6 tbsp plant butter, cold and cubed
- ✓ 1 cup chopped mixed nuts

Directions:

❖ Preheat the oven the 400 F.

❖ Slice off the top of the apples and use a melon baller or spoon to scoop out the cores of the apples. In a bowl, mix the maple syrup, almond flour, date sugar, butter, and nuts. Spoon the mixture into the apples and then bake in the oven for 25 minutes or until the nuts are golden brown on top and the apples soft. Remove the apples from the oven, allow cooling, and serve

82) SUMMER MINT ICE CREAM

Preparation Time: 10 minutes + chilling time		Servings: 4

Ingredients:

- ✓ 2 avocados, pitted
- ✓ 1 ¼ cups coconut cream
- ✓ ½ tsp vanilla extract
- ✓ 2 tbsp erythritol
- ✓ 2 tsp chopped mint leaves

Directions:

❖ Into a blender, spoon the avocado pulps, pour in the coconut cream, vanilla extract, erythritol, and mint leaves. Process until smooth. Pour the mixture into your ice cream maker and freeze according to the manufacturer's instructions. When ready, remove and scoop the ice cream into bowls. Serve

83) TASTY CARDAMOM COCONUT FAT BOMBS

Preparation Time: 10 minutes		Servings: 6

Ingredients:

- ✓ ½ cup grated coconut
- ✓ 3 oz plant butter, softened
- ✓ ¼ tsp green cardamom powder
- ✓ ½ tsp vanilla extract
- ✓ ¼ tsp cinnamon powder

Directions:

❖ Pour the grated coconut into a skillet and roast until lightly brown. Set aside to cool. In a bowl, combine butter, half of the coconut, cardamom, vanilla, and cinnamon. Form balls from the mixture and roll each one in the remaining coconut. Refrigerate until ready to serve

84) HUNGARIAN CINNAMON FAUX RICE PUDDING

Preparation Time: 25 minutes		Servings: 6

Ingredients:

- ✓ 1 ¼ cups coconut cream
- ✓ 1 tsp vanilla extract
- ✓ 1 tsp cinnamon powder
- ✓ 1 cup mashed tofu
- ✓ 2 oz fresh strawberries

Directions:

❖ Pour the coconut cream into a bowl and whisk until a soft peak forms. Mix in the vanilla and cinnamon. Lightly fold in the vegan cottage cheese and refrigerate for 10 to 15 minutes to set. Spoon into serving glasses, top with the strawberries and serve immediately

85) SWEET WHITE CHOCOLATE FUDGE

Preparation Time: 20 minutes + chilling time		Servings: 6

Ingredients:

- ✓ 2 cups coconut cream
- ✓ 1 tsp vanilla extract
- ✓ 3 oz plant butter
- ✓ 3 oz vegan white chocolate
- ✓ Swerve sugar for sprinkling

Directions:

❖ Pour coconut cream and vanilla into a saucepan and bring to a boil over medium heat, then simmer until reduced by half, 15 minutes. Stir in plant butter until the batter is smooth. Chop white chocolate into bits and stir in the cream until melted. Pour the mixture into a baking sheet; chill in the fridge for 3 hours. Cut into squares, sprinkle with swerve sugar, and serve

86) ITALIAN MACEDONIA SALAD WITH COCONUT AND PECANS

Preparation Time: 15 minutes + cooling time		Servings: 4

Ingredients:

- ✓ 1 cup pure coconut cream
- ✓ ½ tsp vanilla extract
- ✓ 2 bananas, cut into chunks
- ✓ 1 ½ cups coconut flakes
- ✓ 4 tbsp toasted pecans, chopped
- ✓ 1 cup pineapple tidbits, drained
- ✓ 1 (11-oz) can mandarin oranges
- ✓ ¾ cup maraschino cherries, stems removed

Directions:

❖ In a medium bowl, mix the coconut cream and vanilla extract until well combined.

❖ In a larger bowl, combine the bananas, coconut flakes, pecans, pineapple, oranges, and cherries until evenly distributed. Pour on the coconut cream mixture and fold well into the salad. Chill in the refrigerator for 1 hour and serve afterward

87) AUTHENTIC BERRY HAZELNUT TRIFLE

Preparation Time: 10 minutes		Servings: 4

Ingredients:

- ✓ 1 ½ ripe avocados
- ✓ ¾ cup coconut cream
- ✓ Zest and juice of ½ a lemon
- ✓ 1 tbsp vanilla extract
- ✓ 3 oz fresh strawberries
- ✓ 2 oz toasted hazelnuts

Directions:

❖ In a bowl, add avocado pulp, coconut cream, lemon zest and juice, and half of the vanilla extract. Mix with an immersion blender. Put the strawberries and remaining vanilla in another bowl and use a fork to mash the fruits. In a tall glass, alternate layering the cream and strawberry mixtures. Drop a few hazelnuts on each and serve the dessert immediately

88) VEGETARIAN AVOCADO TRUFFLES WITH CHOCOLATE COATING

Preparation Time: 5 minutes		Servings: 6

Ingredients:

- ✓ 1 ripe avocado, pitted
- ✓ ½ tsp vanilla extract
- ✓ ½ tsp lemon zest
- ✓ 5 oz dairy-free dark chocolate
- ✓ 1 tbsp coconut oil
- ✓ 1 tbsp unsweetened cocoa powder

Directions:

❖ Scoop the pulp of the avocado into a bowl and mix with the vanilla using an immersion blender. Stir in the lemon zest and a pinch of salt. Pour the chocolate and coconut oil into a safe microwave bowl and melt in the microwave for 1 minute. Add to the avocado mixture and stir. Allow cooling to firm up a bit. Form balls out of the mix. Roll each ball in the cocoa powder and serve immediately

89) DELICIOUS VANILLA BERRY TARTS

Preparation Time: 35 minutes + cooling time		Servings: 4

Ingredients:

- ✓ 4 tbsp flaxseed powder
- ✓ 1/3 cup whole-wheat flour
- ✓ ½ tsp salt
- ✓ ¼ cup plant butter, crumbled
- ✓ 3 tbsp pure malt syrup
- ✓ 6 oz cashew cream
- ✓ 6 tbsp pure date sugar
- ✓ ¾ tsp vanilla extract
- ✓ 1 cup mixed frozen berries

Directions:

❖ Preheat oven to 350 F and grease mini pie pans with cooking spray. In a bowl, mix flaxseed powder with 12 tbsp water and allow soaking for 5 minutes. In a large bowl, combine flour and salt. Add in butter and whisk until crumbly. Pour in the vegan "flax egg" and malt syrup and mix until smooth dough forms. Flatten the dough on a flat surface, cover with plastic wrap, and refrigerate for 1 hour.

❖ Dust a working surface with some flour, remove the dough onto the surface, and using a rolling pin, flatten the dough into a 1-inch diameter circle. Use a large cookie cutter, cut out rounds of the dough and fit into the pie pans. Use a knife to trim the edges of the pan. Lay a parchment paper on the dough cups, pour on some baking beans, and bake in the oven until golden brown, 15-20 minutes. Remove the pans from the oven, pour out the baking beans, and allow cooling. In a bowl, mix cashew cream, date sugar, and vanilla extract. Divide the mixture into the tart cups and top with berries. Serve

90) ITALIAN AROMATIC MILLET BOWL

Preparation Time: 20 minutes		Servings: 3

Ingredients:

- ✓ 1 cup water
- ✓ 1 ½ cups coconut milk
- ✓ 1 cup millet, rinsed and drained
- ✓ 1/4 tsp crystallized ginger
- ✓ 1/4 tsp ground cinnamon
- ✓ A pinch of grated nutmeg
- ✓ A pinch of Himalayan salt
- ✓ 2 tbsp maple syrup

Directions:

❖ Place the water, milk, millet, crystallized ginger cinnamon, nutmeg and salt in a saucepan; bring to a boil.

❖ Turn the heat to a simmer and let it cook for about 20 minutes; fluff the millet with a fork and spoon into individual bowls.

❖ Serve with maple syrup. Enjoy

91) SPICY HARISSA BULGUR BOWL

Preparation Time: 25 minutes

Servings: 4

Ingredients:

- ✓ 1 cup bulgur wheat
- ✓ 1 ½ cups vegetable broth
- ✓ 2 cups sweet corn kernels, thawed
- ✓ 1 cup canned kidney beans, drained
- ✓ 1 red onion, thinly sliced
- ✓ 1 garlic clove, minced
- ✓ Sea salt and ground black pepper, to taste
- ✓ 1/4 cup harissa paste
- ✓ 1 tbsp lemon juice
- ✓ 1 tbsp white vinegar
- ✓ 1/4 cup extra-virgin olive oil
- ✓ 1/4 cup fresh parsley leaves, roughly chopped

Directions:

- ❖ In a deep saucepan, bring the bulgur wheat and vegetable broth to a simmer; let it cook, covered, for 12 to 13 minutes.
- ❖ Let it stand for 5 to 10 minutes and fluff your bulgur with a fork.
- ❖ Add the remaining ingredients to the cooked bulgur wheat; serve warm or at room temperature. Enjoy

92) EXOTIC COCONUT QUINOA PUDDING

Preparation Time: 20 minutes

Servings: 3

Ingredients:

- ✓ 1 cup water
- ✓ 1 cup coconut milk
- ✓ 1 cup quinoa
- ✓ A pinch of kosher salt
- ✓ A pinch of ground allspice
- ✓ 1/2 tsp cinnamon
- ✓ 1/2 tsp vanilla extract
- ✓ 4 tbsp agave syrup
- ✓ 1/2 cup coconut flakes

Directions:

- ❖ Place the water, coconut milk, quinoa, salt, ground allspice, cinnamon and vanilla extract in a saucepan.
- ❖ Bring it to a boil over medium-high heat. Turn the heat to a simmer and let it cook for about 20 minutes; fluff with a fork and add in the agave syrup.
- ❖ Divide between three serving bowls and garnish with coconut flakes. Enjoy

93) ITALIAN CREMINI MUSHROOM RISOTTO

Preparation Time: 20 minutes

Servings: 3

Ingredients:

- ✓ 3 tbsp vegan butter
- ✓ 1 tsp garlic, minced
- ✓ 1 tsp thyme
- ✓ 1 pound Cremini mushrooms, sliced
- ✓ 1 ½ cups white rice
- ✓ 2 ½ cups vegetable broth
- ✓ 1/4 cup dry sherry wine
- ✓ Kosher salt and ground black pepper, to taste
- ✓ 3 tbsp fresh scallions, thinly sliced

Directions:

- ❖ In a saucepan, melt the vegan butter over a moderately high flame. Cook the garlic and thyme for about 1 minute or until aromatic.
- ❖ Add in the mushrooms and continue to sauté until they release the liquid or about 3 minutes.
- ❖ Add in the rice, vegetable broth and sherry wine. Bring to a boil; immediately turn the heat to a gentle simmer.
- ❖ Cook for about 15 minutes or until all the liquid has absorbed. Fluff the rice with a fork, season with salt and pepper and garnish with fresh scallions. Enjoy

94) BEST HOMEMADE CHOCOLATES WITH COCONUT AND RAISINS

Preparation Time: 10 minutes + chilling time		Servings: 20

Ingredients:

- ✓ 1/2 cup cacao butter, melted
- ✓ 1/3 cup peanut butter
- ✓ 1/4 cup agave syrup
- ✓ A pinch of grated nutmeg
- ✓ A pinch of coarse salt
- ✓ 1/2 tsp vanilla extract
- ✓ 1 cup dried coconut, shredded
- ✓ 6 ounces dark chocolate, chopped
- ✓ 3 ounces raisins

Directions:

- ❖ Thoroughly combine all the ingredients, except for the chocolate, in a mixing bowl.
- ❖ Spoon the mixture into molds. Leave to set hard in a cool place.
- ❖ Melt the dark chocolate in your microwave. Pour in the melted chocolate until the fillings are covered. Leave to set hard in a cool place.
- ❖ Enjoy

95) SIMPLE MOCHA FUDGE

Preparation Time: 1 hour 10 minutes		Servings: 20

Ingredients:

- ✓ 1 cup cookies, crushed
- ✓ 1/2 cup almond butter
- ✓ 1/4 cup agave nectar
- ✓ 6 ounces dark chocolate, broken into chunks
- ✓ 1 tsp instant coffee
- ✓ A pinch of grated nutmeg
- ✓ A pinch of salt

Directions:

- ❖ Line a large baking sheet with parchment paper.
- ❖ Melt the chocolate in your microwave and add in the remaining ingredients; stir to combine well.
- ❖ Scrape the batter into a parchment-lined baking sheet. Place it in your freezer for at least 1 hour to set.
- ❖ Cut into squares and serve. Enjoy

96) EAST ALMOND AND CHOCOLATE CHIP BARS

Preparation Time: 40 minutes		Servings: 10

Ingredients:

- ✓ 1/2 cup almond butter
- ✓ 1/4 cup coconut oil, melted
- ✓ 1/4 cup agave syrup
- ✓ 1 tsp vanilla extract
- ✓ 1/4 tsp sea salt
- ✓ 1/4 tsp grated nutmeg
- ✓ 1/2 tsp ground cinnamon
- ✓ 2 cups almond flour
- ✓ 1/4 cup flaxseed meal
- ✓ 1 cup vegan chocolate, cut into chunks
- ✓ 1 1/3 cups almonds, ground
- ✓ 2 tbsp cacao powder
- ✓ 1/4 cup agave syrup

Directions:

- ❖ In a mixing bowl, thoroughly combine the almond butter, coconut oil, 1/4 cup of agave syrup, vanilla, salt, nutmeg and cinnamon.
- ❖ Gradually stir in the almond flour and flaxseed meal and stir to combine. Add in the chocolate chunks and stir again.
- ❖ In a small mixing bowl, combine the almonds, cacao powder and agave syrup. Now, spread the ganache onto the cake. Freeze for about 30 minutes, cut into bars and serve well chilled. Enjoy

97) ALMOND BUTTER COOKIES

Preparation Time: 45 minutes		Servings: 10

Ingredients:

- ✓ 3/4 cup all-purpose flour
- ✓ 1/2 tsp baking soda
- ✓ 1/4 tsp kosher salt
- ✓ 1 flax egg
- ✓ 1/4 cup coconut oil, at room temperature
- ✓ 2 tbsp almond milk
- ✓ 1/2 cup brown sugar
- ✓ 1/2 cup almond butter
- ✓ 1/2 tsp ground cinnamon
- ✓ 1/2 tsp vanilla

Directions:

- ❖ In a mixing bowl, combine the flour, baking soda and salt.
- ❖ In another bowl, combine the flax egg, coconut oil, almond milk, sugar, almond butter, cinnamon and vanilla. Stir the wet mixture into the dry ingredients and stir until well combined.
- ❖ Place the batter in your refrigerator for about 30 minutes. Shape the batter into small cookies and arrange them on a parchment-lined cookie pan.
- ❖ Bake in the preheated oven at 350 degrees F for approximately 12 minutes. Transfer the pan to a wire rack to cool at room temperature. Enjoy

98) AMERICAN PEANUT BUTTER OATMEAL BARS

Preparation Time: 25 minutes		Servings: 20

Ingredients:

- ✓ 1 cup vegan butter
- ✓ 3/4 cup coconut sugar
- ✓ 2 tbsp applesauce
- ✓ 1 ¾ cups old-fashioned oats
- ✓ 1 tsp baking soda
- ✓ A pinch of sea salt
- ✓ A pinch of grated nutmeg
- ✓ 1 tsp pure vanilla extract
- ✓ 1 cup oat flour
- ✓ 1 cup all-purpose flour

Directions:

- ❖ Begin by preheating your oven to 350 degrees F.
- ❖ In a mixing bowl, thoroughly combine the dry ingredients. In another bowl, combine the wet ingredients.
- ❖ Then, stir the wet mixture into the dry ingredients; mix to combine well.
- ❖ Spread the batter mixture in a parchment-lined square baking pan. Bake in the preheated oven for about 20 minutes. Enjoy

99) SPECIAL VANILLA HALVAH FUDGE

Preparation Time: 10 minutes + chilling time		Servings: 16

Ingredients:

- ✓ 1/2 cup cocoa butter
- ✓ 1/2 cup tahini
- ✓ 8 dates, pitted
- ✓ 1/4 tsp ground cloves
- ✓ A pinch of grated nutmeg
- ✓ A pinch coarse salt
- ✓ 1 tsp vanilla extract

Directions:

- ❖ Line a square baking pan with parchment paper.
- ❖ Mix the ingredients until everything is well incorporated.
- ❖ Scrape the batter into the parchment-lined pan. Place in your freezer until ready to serve. Enjoy

100) HEALTHY RAW CHOCOLATE MANGO PIE

Preparation Time: 10 minutes + chilling time | | **Servings: 16**

Ingredients:

- ✓ Avocado layer:
- ✓ 3 ripe avocados, pitted and peeled
- ✓ A pinch of sea salt
- ✓ A pinch of ground anise
- ✓ 1/2 tsp vanilla paste
- ✓ 2 tbsp coconut milk
- ✓ 5 tbsp agave syrup
- ✓ 1/3 cup cocoa powder
- ✓ Crema layer:
- ✓ 1/3 cup almond butter
- ✓ 1/2 cup coconut cream
- ✓ 1 medium mango, peeled
- ✓ 1/2 coconut flakes
- ✓ 2 tbsp agave syrup

Directions:

- ❖ In your food processor, blend the avocado layer until smooth and uniform, reserve.
- ❖ Then, blend the other layer in a separate bowl. Spoon the layers in a lightly oiled baking pan.
- ❖ Transfer the cake to your freezer for about 3 hours. Store in your freezer. Enjoy

101) FROZEN CHOCOLATE N'ICE CREAM

Preparation Time: 10 minutes | | **Servings: 1**

Ingredients:

- ✓ 2 frozen bananas, peeled and sliced
- ✓ 2 tbsp coconut milk
- ✓ 1 tsp carob powder
- ✓ 1 tsp cocoa powder
- ✓ A pinch of grated nutmeg
- ✓ 1/8 tsp ground cardamom
- ✓ 1/8 tsp ground cinnamon
- ✓ 1 tbsp chocolate curls

Directions:

- ❖ Place all the ingredients in the bowl of your food processor or high-speed blender.
- ❖ Blitz the ingredients until creamy or until your desired consistency is achieved.
- ❖ Serve immediately or store in your freezer.
- ❖ Enjoy

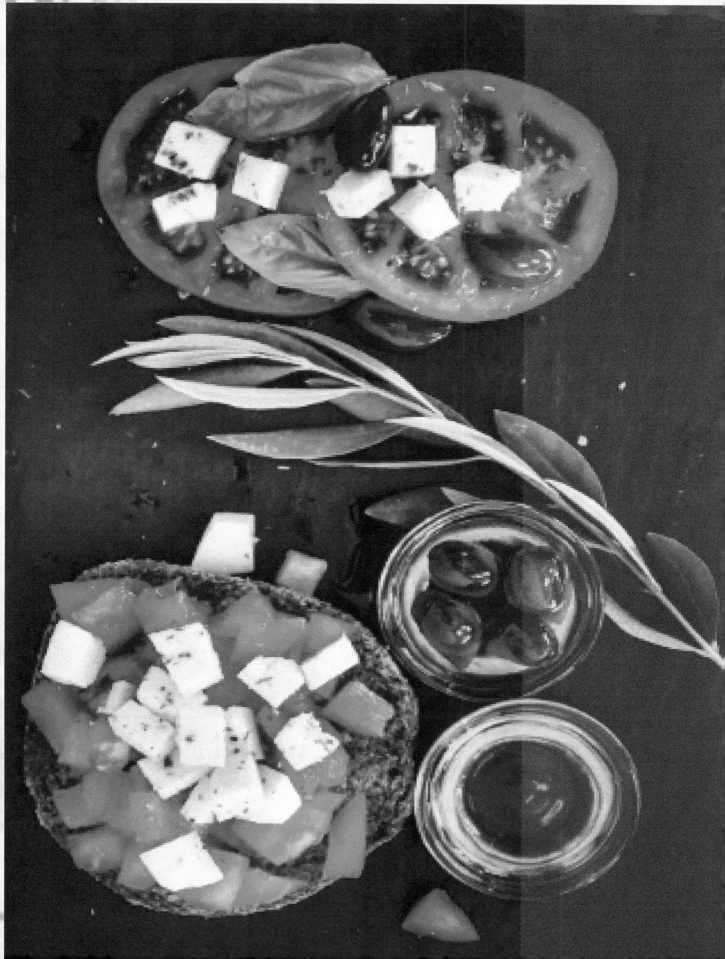

The Best Exercises to <u>SCULPT</u> your Body

1) 3 series X 30 **CRUNCHES** (Stop for 30" from each series)

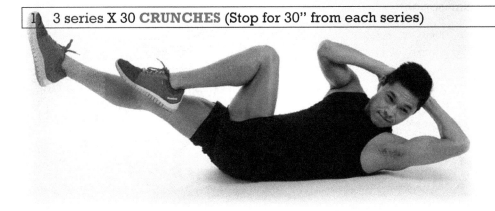

2) 3 series X 30" **PLANK** (Stop for 30" from each series)

3) 3 series X 20
CROSS FIT CRUNCHES

(Stop for 10" from each series)

Start in crunch position with legs up. Take a 5kg ball and move on the left side your arms. Move your arms to the other side. Keep the legs up!

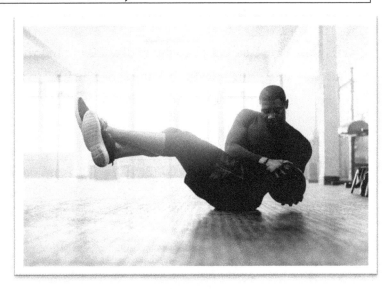

4) 3 series X 20 **CROSS BODY** (Stop for 10" from each series)

In plank position up your left leg and cross it with the right side. Repeat with the other side.

5) 3 series X 30" **PLANK SIDEWALK** (Stop for 10" from each series)

In plank position, move yourself: the first step with left leg on the left; then the second step with the right leg on the left. Make 3 complete steps and return at the beginning place, making steps one by one on the right.

6) 3 series X 30 **DIAMOND PRESS-UPS**

   (Stop for 30" from each series)

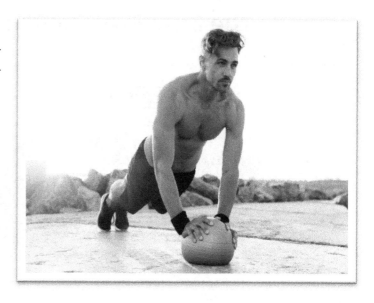

1) 3 series X 30 **LEG TRAX** (Stop for 10" from each series)

Fix your Exercise Bands to the wall at 30 cm height from the down. Lie down on the floor and link the band with your legs. Put perpendicular to the roof your left-right and move it to touch the floor. Keep it rigid and return at the beginning. Repeat with the right leg.

2) 3 series X 20 **SQUATS** (Stop for 30" from each series)

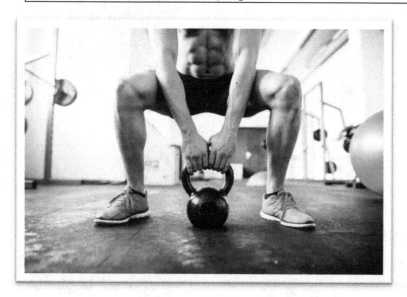

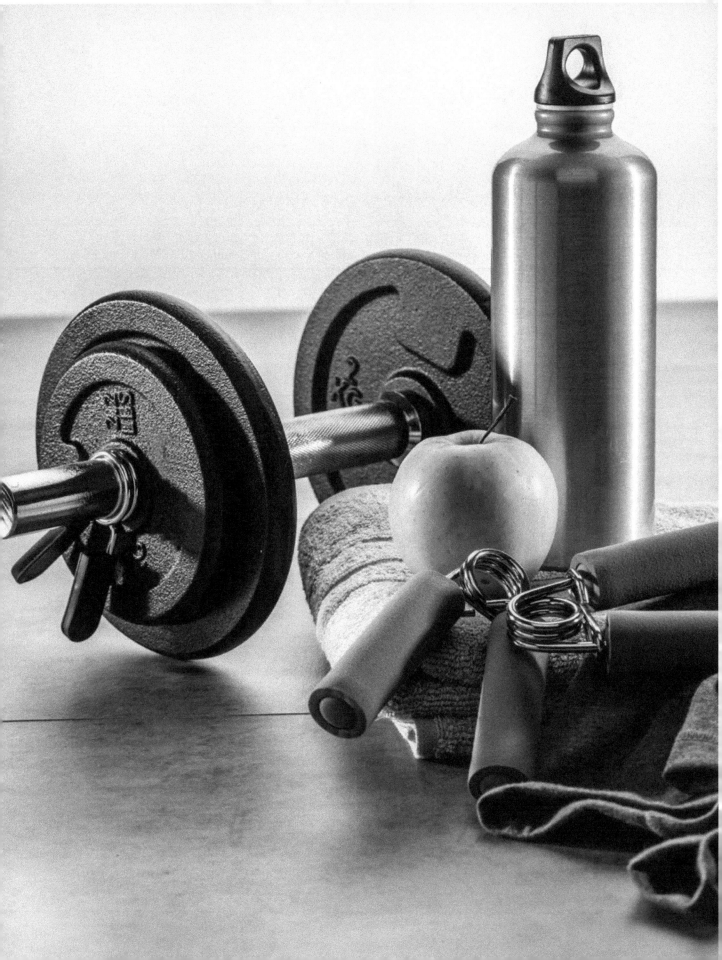

Bibliography

FROM THE SAME AUTHOR

THE VEGETARIAN DIET *Cookbook* - 100+ Easy-to-Follow Recipes for Beginners! TASTE Yourself with the Most Vibrant Plant-Based Cuisine Meals!

THE VEGETARIAN DIET FOR ATHLETES *Cookbook* - The Best Recipes for Athletic Performance and Muscle Growth! More Than 100 High-Protein Plant-Based Meals to Maintain a Perfect Body!

THE VEGETARIAN DIET FOR BEGINNERS *Cookbook* - 100+ Super Easy Recipes to Start a Healthier Lifestyle! The Best Recipes You Need to Jump into the Tastiest Plant-Based World!

THE VEGETARIAN DIET FOR MEN *Cookbook* - The Best 100 Recipes to Stay FIT! Sculpt Your Abs Before Summer with the Healthiest Plant-Based Meals!

THE VEGETARIAN DIET FOR WOMEN *Cookbook* - The Best 100 recipes to stay TONE and HEALTHY! Reboot your Metabolism before Summer with the Tastiest and Lightest Plant-Based Meals!

THE VEGETARIAN DIET FOR KIDS *Cookbook* - The Best 100 recipes for children, tested BY Kids FOR Kids! Jump into the Plant-Based World to Stay Healthy HAVING FUN!

THE VEGETARIAN DIET FOR WOMEN OVER 50 *Cookbook* - The Best Plant-Based Recipes to Restart Your Metabolism! Maintain the Right Hormonal Balance and Lose Weight with More Than 100 Light and Healthy Recipes!

THE VEGETARIAN DIET FOT MEN OVER 50 *Cookbook* - The Best Recipes to Restart Your Metabolism! Stay Healthy with More than 100 Easy and Mouthwatering Recipes!

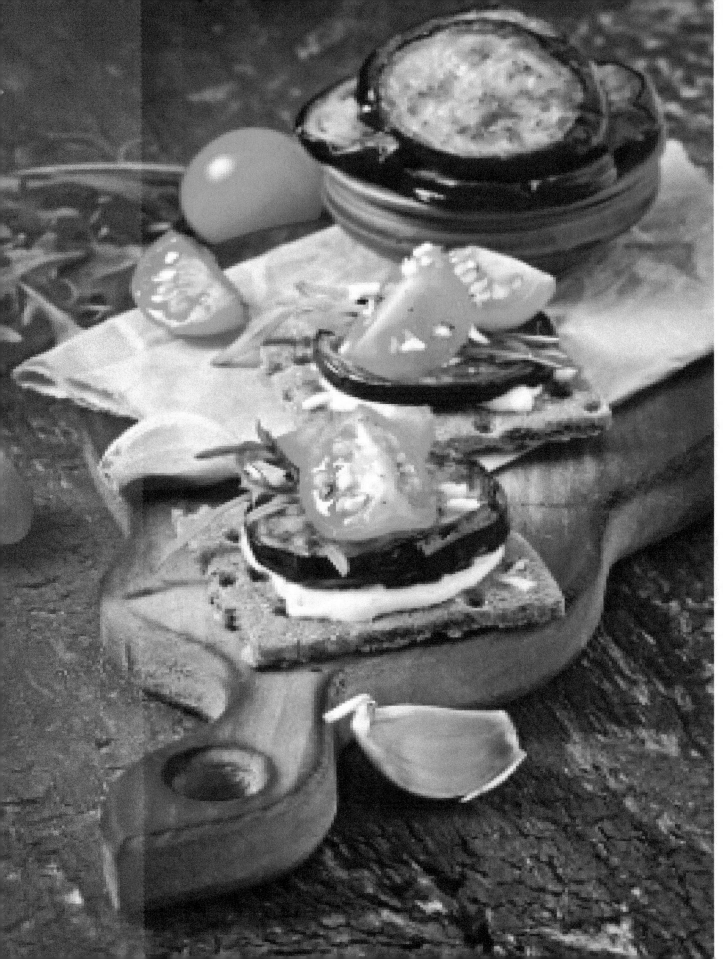

Conclusion

Thanks for reading "Vegetarian Diet for Men *Cookbook*"!

Follow the right habits it is essential to have a healthy Lifestyle, and the Vegetarian diet is the best solution!

I hope you liked this Cookbook!

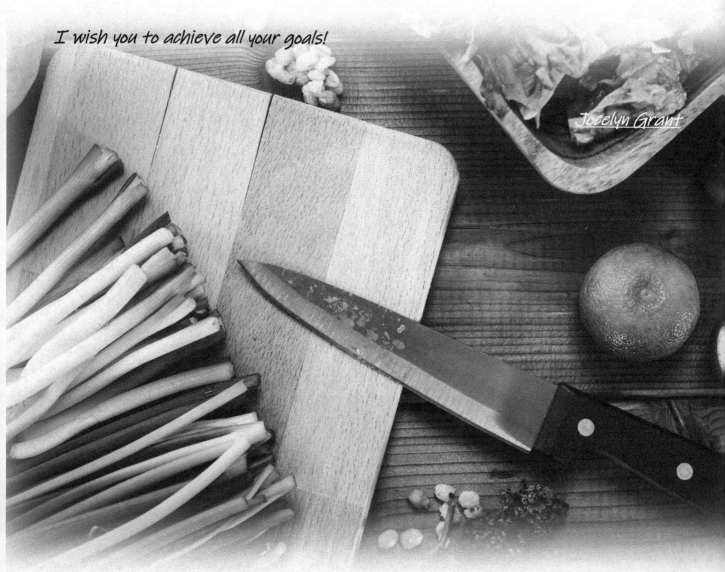

I wish you to achieve all your goals!

Jocelyn Grant

CPSIA information can be obtained
at www.ICGtesting.com
Printed in the USA
BVHW011030290421
606130BV00006B/1160